Schick

Anatomy Atlas

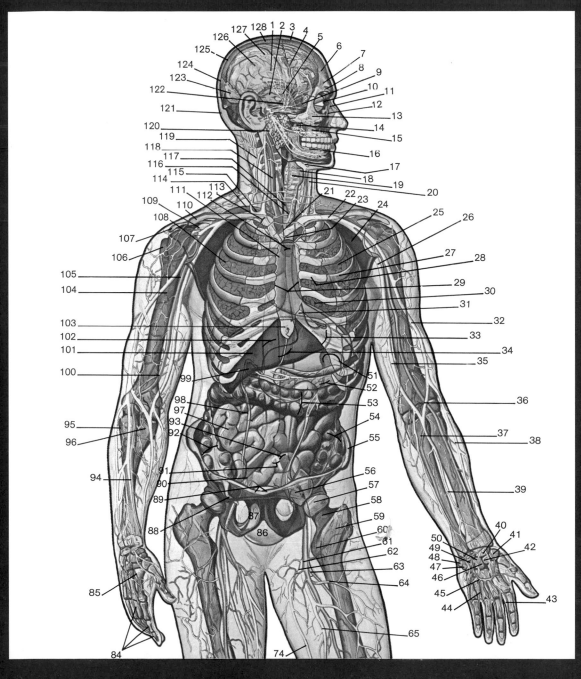

American Map® Corporation

Contents

NS1 **SKELETON AND ARTERIES**
Front view, full figure: main
arteries, pressure points.

NS2 **EYE-VISION**
Normal, myopic, hyperopic,
compensating lenses.

NS3 **SKIN**
Cross-section, sensory organs.

NS4 **HEART**
With supplementary
figures.

NS5 **DIGESTIVE SYSTEM**
General.

NS6 **INTESTINAL VILLUS &
DIGESTIVE DISORDERS**

NS7 **RESPIRATORY TRACT**
General.

NS8 **NERVOUS CONTROL OF
RESPIRATION AND SYMPTOMS
OF INFECTIONS**

NS9 **EAR**
Inner and outer.

NS10 **KIDNEYS**
In position, cross-sections,
disorders.

NS11 **DEVELOPMENT OF THE
EMBRYO**
From cell to 8th week.

NS12 **FEMALE REPRODUCTIVE
ORGANS**
Includes pregnancy at term.

NS13 **MALE REPRODUCTIVE
ORGANS**

NS14 **EYE**
Protective mechanism.

NS15 **EYE**
Sight as a function of the brain.

NS16 **DEVELOPMENT OF THE
BLOOD CELLS**
Origin, structure.

NS17 **BLOOD CELLS**
Structure, function, groups,
counts.

NS18 **DISEASES OF THE BLOOD
CELLS**

NS19 **HUMAN BODY**
Front view, full figure: all
organs, blood circulation.

NS20 **THROAT**
Section, larynx and pharynx,
vocal cords, pathological con-
ditions.

NS21 **HUMAN BODY**
Back view, full figure: bones,
muscles, system of nerves.

NS22 **ENDOCRINE GLANDS**
Relative size and correct position
in body.

NS23 **ENDOCRINE SYSTEM**
Enlarged view and diagram of
interrelations: schematic chart.

NS24 **LYMPHATIC SYSTEM**
General.

NS25 **LYMPHATIC SYSTEM**
Enlarged sections, nodes,
vessels.

NS26 **BRAIN**
Sagittal section: head, neck,
chest; schematic connection
between nervous system and
heart.

NS27 **BRAIN**
Median sagittal and horizontal
sections, spinal cord, base of
brain.

NS28 **TISSUES**
Types of epithelial, muscular,
and nervous tissues.

NS29 **TISSUES**
Twelve types of connective
tissues.

NS30 **AUTONOMIC NERVOUS
SYSTEM**

INDEX

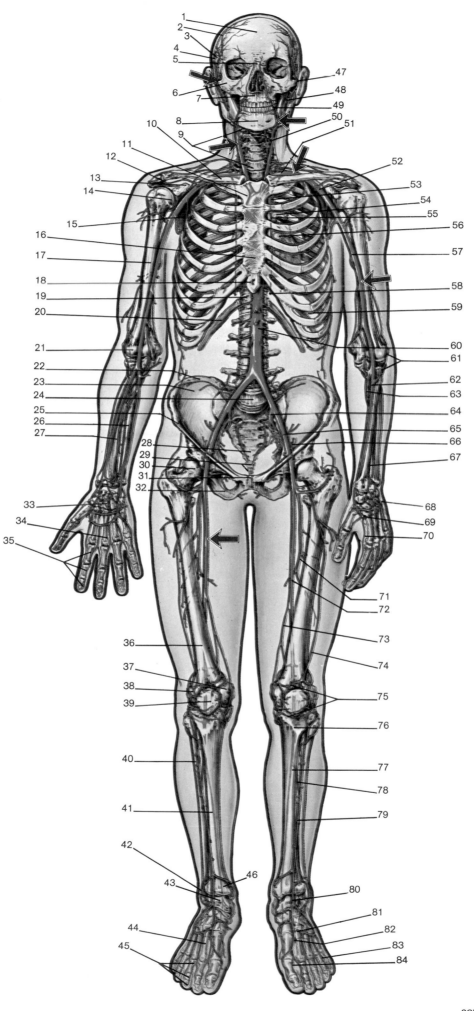

SCHICK-COLORPRINT® ANATOMY CHART
SKELETON AND ARTERIES
No. NS1 © 1988 AMERICAN MAP CORP.

SKELETON AND ARTERIES

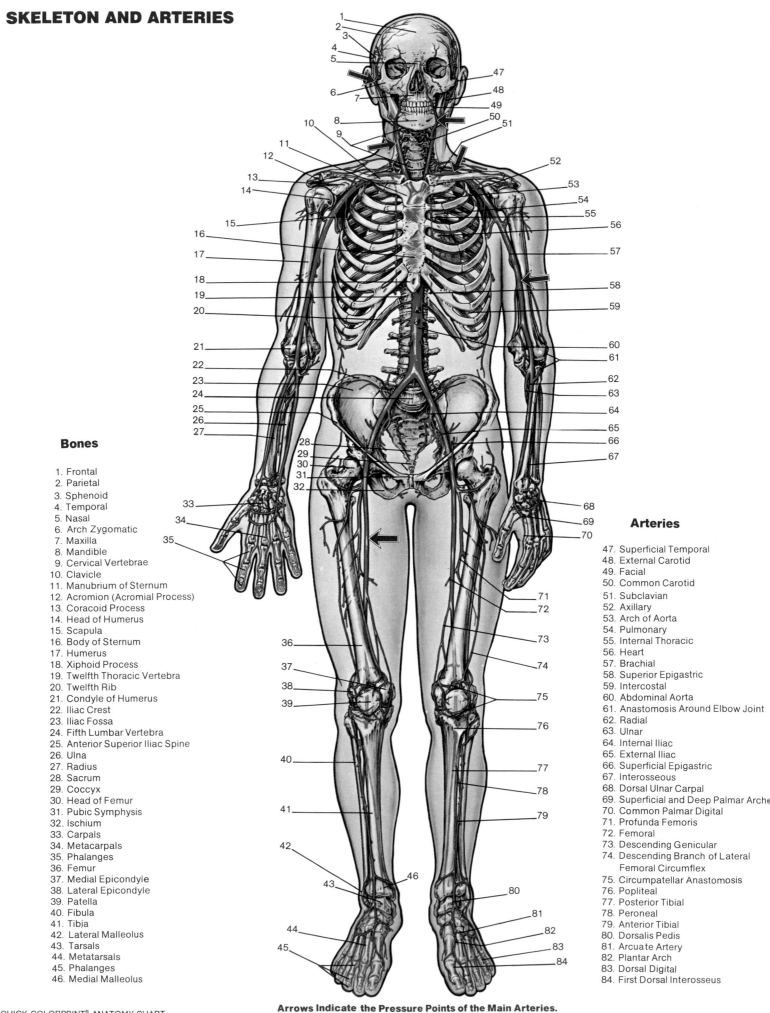

Bones

1. Frontal
2. Parietal
3. Sphenoid
4. Temporal
5. Nasal
6. Arch Zygomatic
7. Maxilla
8. Mandible
9. Cervical Vertebrae
10. Clavicle
11. Manubrium of Sternum
12. Acromion (Acromial Process)
13. Coracoid Process
14. Head of Humerus
15. Scapula
16. Body of Sternum
17. Humerus
18. Xiphoid Process
19. Twelfth Thoracic Vertebra
20. Twelfth Rib
21. Condyle of Humerus
22. Iliac Crest
23. Iliac Fossa
24. Fifth Lumbar Vertebra
25. Anterior Superior Iliac Spine
26. Ulna
27. Radius
28. Sacrum
29. Coccyx
30. Head of Femur
31. Pubic Symphysis
32. Ischium
33. Carpals
34. Metacarpals
35. Phalanges
36. Femur
37. Medial Epicondyle
38. Lateral Epicondyle
39. Patella
40. Fibula
41. Tibia
42. Lateral Malleolus
43. Tarsals
44. Metatarsals
45. Phalanges
46. Medial Malleolus

Arteries

47. Superficial Temporal
48. External Carotid
49. Facial
50. Common Carotid
51. Subclavian
52. Axillary
53. Arch of Aorta
54. Pulmonary
55. Internal Thoracic
56. Heart
57. Brachial
58. Superior Epigastric
59. Intercostal
60. Abdominal Aorta
61. Anastomosis Around Elbow Joint
62. Radial
63. Ulnar
64. Internal Iliac
65. External Iliac
66. Superficial Epigastric
67. Interosseous
68. Dorsal Ulnar Carpal
69. Superficial and Deep Palmar Arch
70. Common Palmar Digital
71. Profunda Femoris
72. Femoral
73. Descending Genicular
74. Descending Branch of Lateral Femoral Circumflex
75. Circumpatellar Anastomosis
76. Popliteal
77. Posterior Tibial
78. Peroneal
79. Anterior Tibial
80. Dorsalis Pedis
81. Arcuate Artery
82. Plantar Arch
83. Dorsal Digital
84. First Dorsal Interosseus

Arrows Indicate the Pressure Points of the Main Arteries.

SCHICK-COLORPRINT® ANATOMY CHART
SKELETON AND ARTERIES
No. NS1 © 1988 AMERICAN MAP CORP.

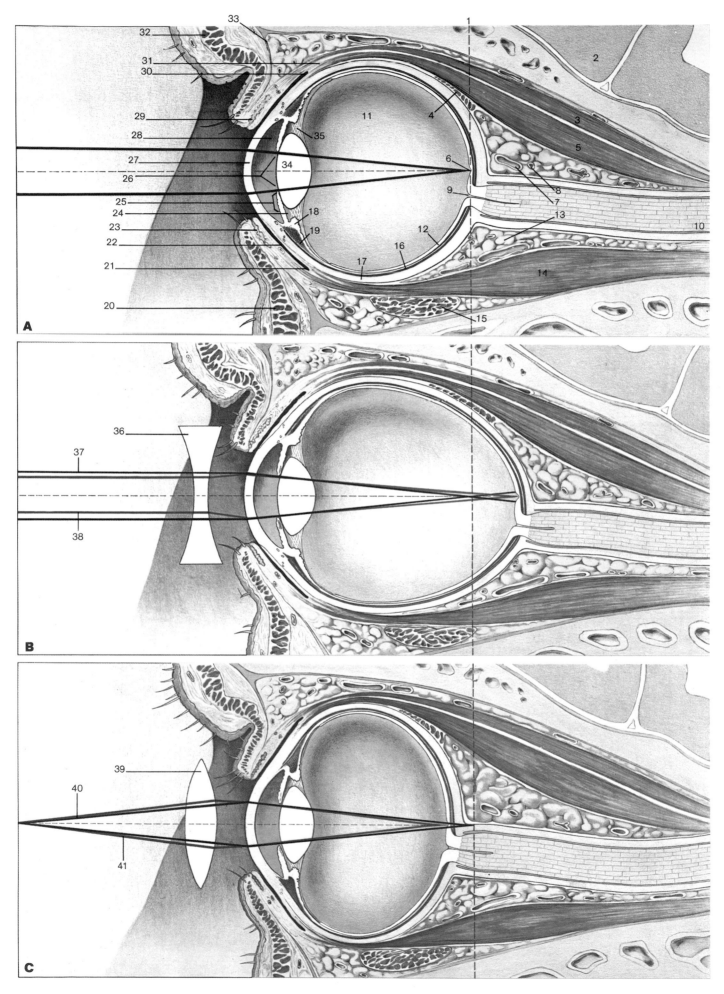

EYE - Vision

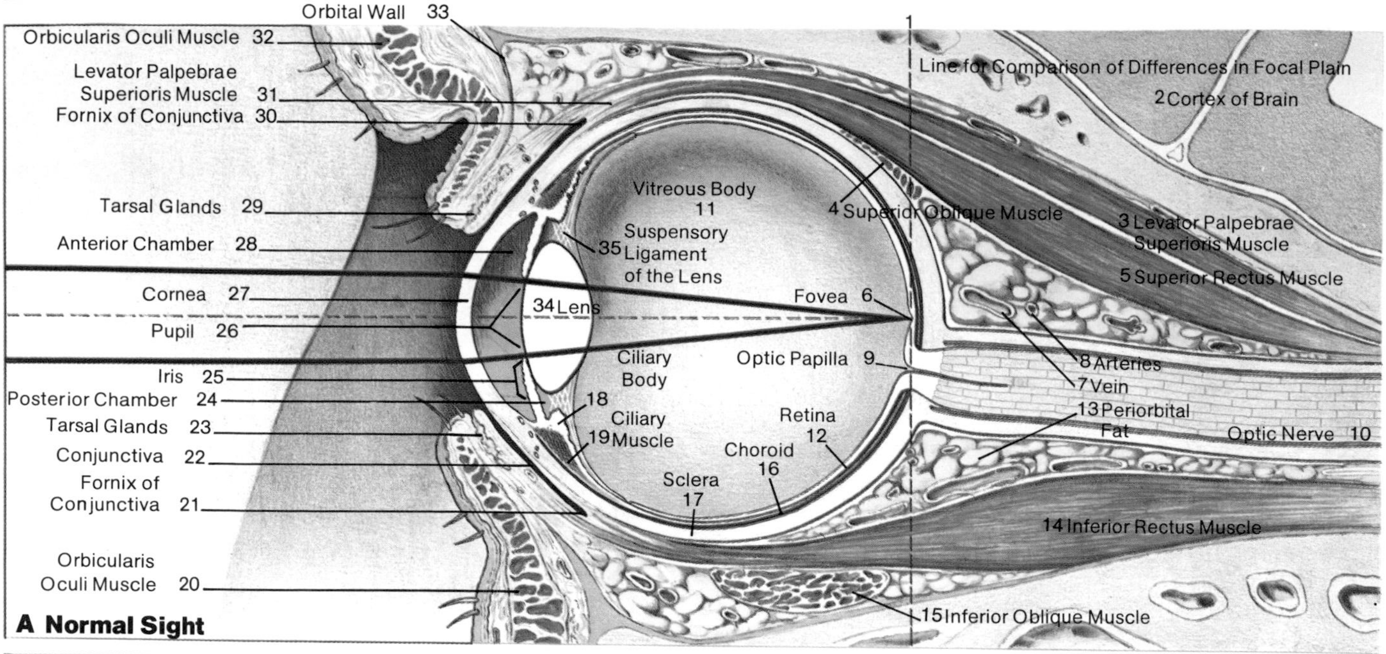

A Normal Sight

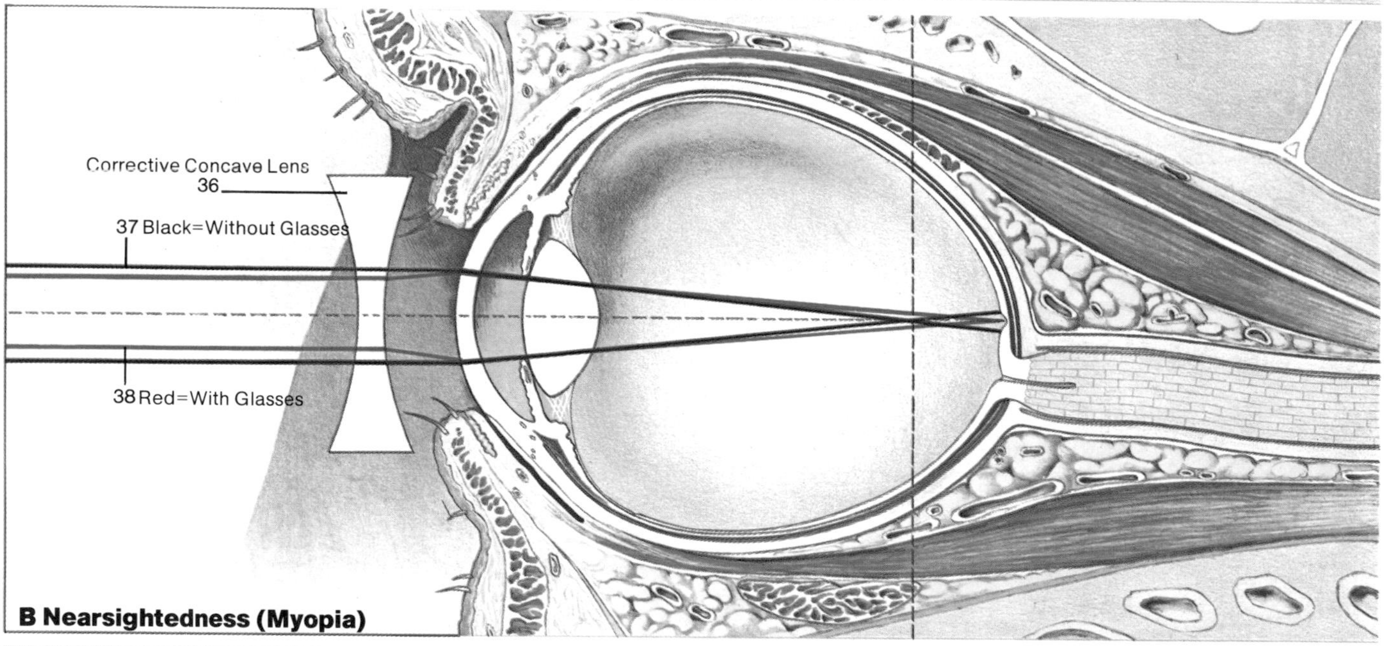

Orbital Wall 33
Orbiculars Oculi Muscle 32
Levator Palpebrae Superioris Muscle 31
Fornix of Conjunctiva 30
Tarsal Glands 29
Anterior Chamber 28
Cornea 27
Pupil 26
Iris 25
Posterior Chamber 24
Tarsal Glands 23
Conjunctiva 22
Fornix of Conjunctiva 21
Orbicularis Oculi Muscle 20

Vitreous Body 11
Suspensory Ligament of the Lens 35
34 Lens
Ciliary Body
18
Ciliary Muscle 19
Sclera 17

Fovea 6
Optic Papilla 9
Retina 12
Choroid 16

Line for Comparison of Differences in Focal Plain
1
2 Cortex of Brain
4 Superior Oblique Muscle
3 Levator Palpebrae Superioris Muscle
5 Superior Rectus Muscle
8 Arteries
7 Vein
13 Periorbital Fat
Optic Nerve 10
14 Inferior Rectus Muscle
15 Inferior Oblique Muscle

B Nearsightedness (Myopia)

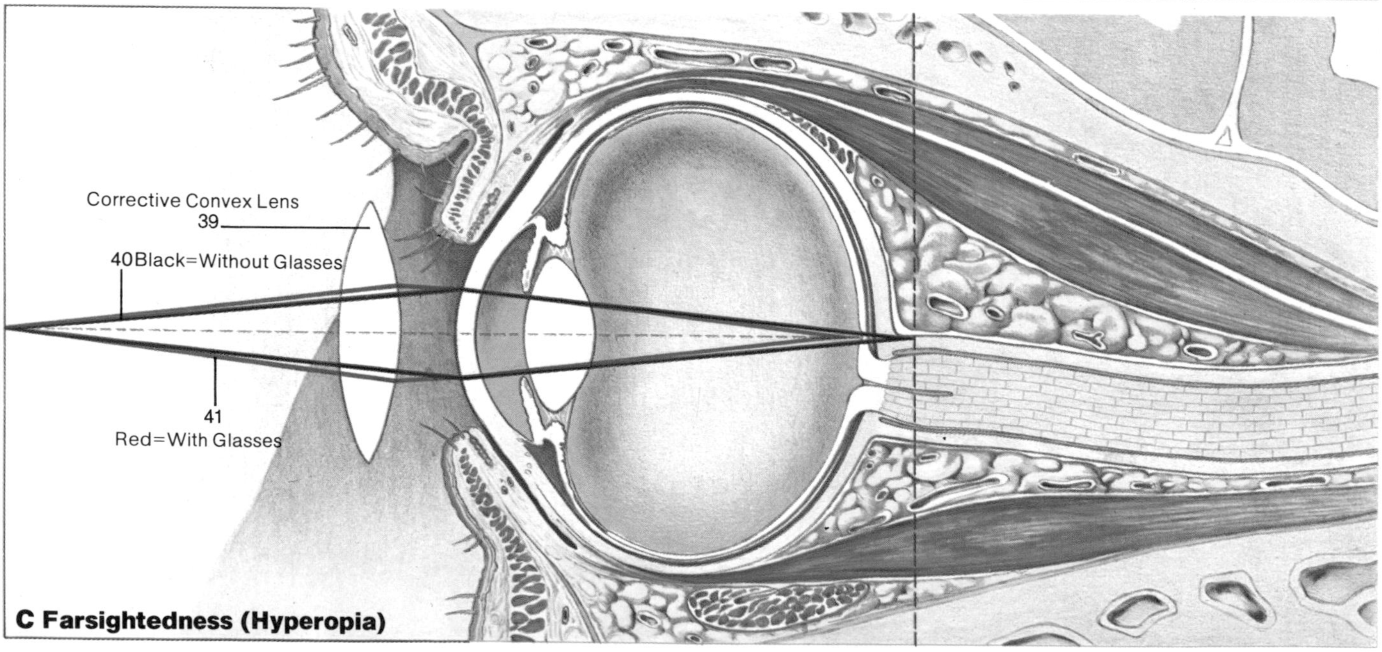

Corrective Concave Lens 36
37 Black=Without Glasses
38 Red=With Glasses

C Farsightedness (Hyperopia)

Corrective Convex Lens 39
40 Black=Without Glasses
41 Red=With Glasses

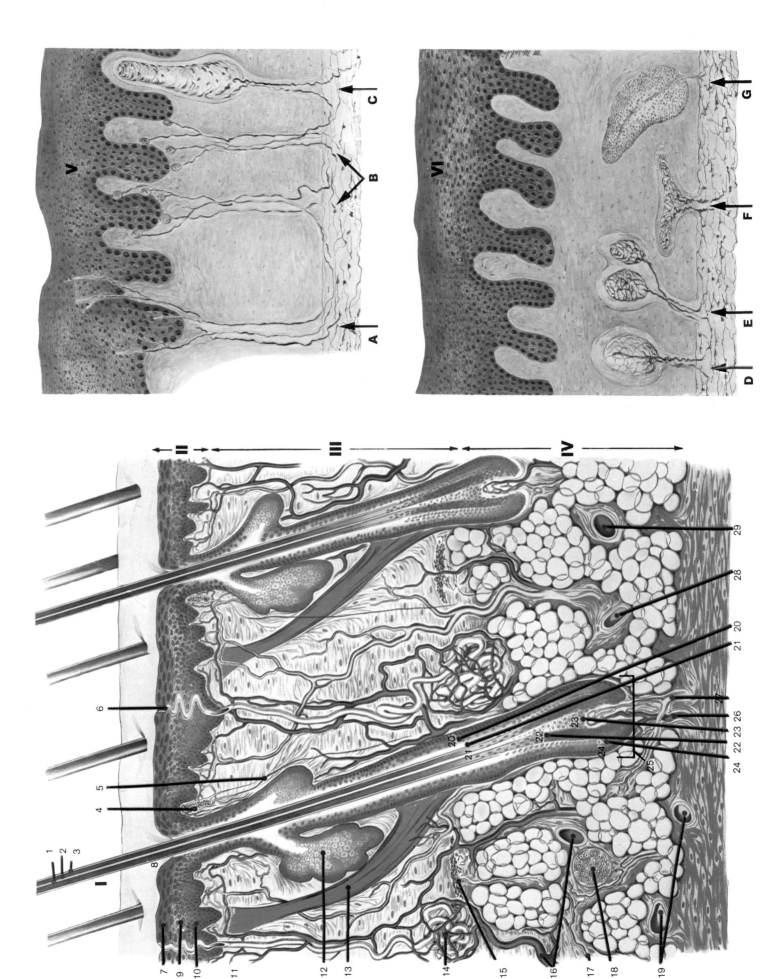

SKIN

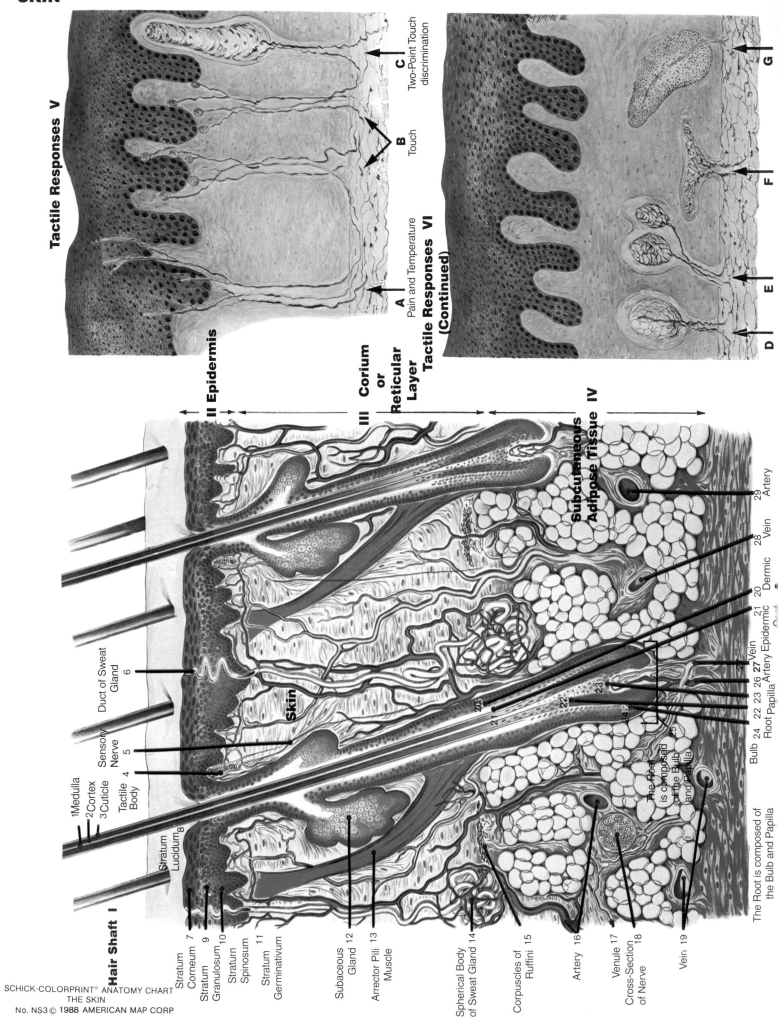

Tactile Responses V

C — Two-Point Touch discrimination

B — Touch

A — Pain and Temperature

Tactile Responses VI (Continued)

G

F

E

D

II Epidermis

III Corium or Reticular Layer

IV Subcutaneous Adipose Tissue

Hair Shaft I

1 Medulla
2 Cortex
3 Cuticle
Tactile Body 4
Sensory Nerve 5
Duct of Sweat Gland 6
Stratum Lucidum 8

Stratum Corneum 7
Stratum Granulosum 9
10
Stratum Spinosum 11
Stratum Germinativum

Subaceous Gland 12
Arrector Pili Muscle 13

Skin

Spherical Body of Sweat Gland 14
Corpuscles of Ruffini 15
Artery 16
Venule 17
Cross-Section of Nerve 18
Vein 19

The Root is composed of the Bulb and Papilla

Bulb 24 22 23 26 **27** Vein
Root Papilla Artery Epidermic

20 Dermic
21 Epidermic
28 Vein
29 Artery

SCHICK-COLORPRINT® ANATOMY CHART
THE SKIN
No. NS3 © 1988 AMERICAN MAP CORP

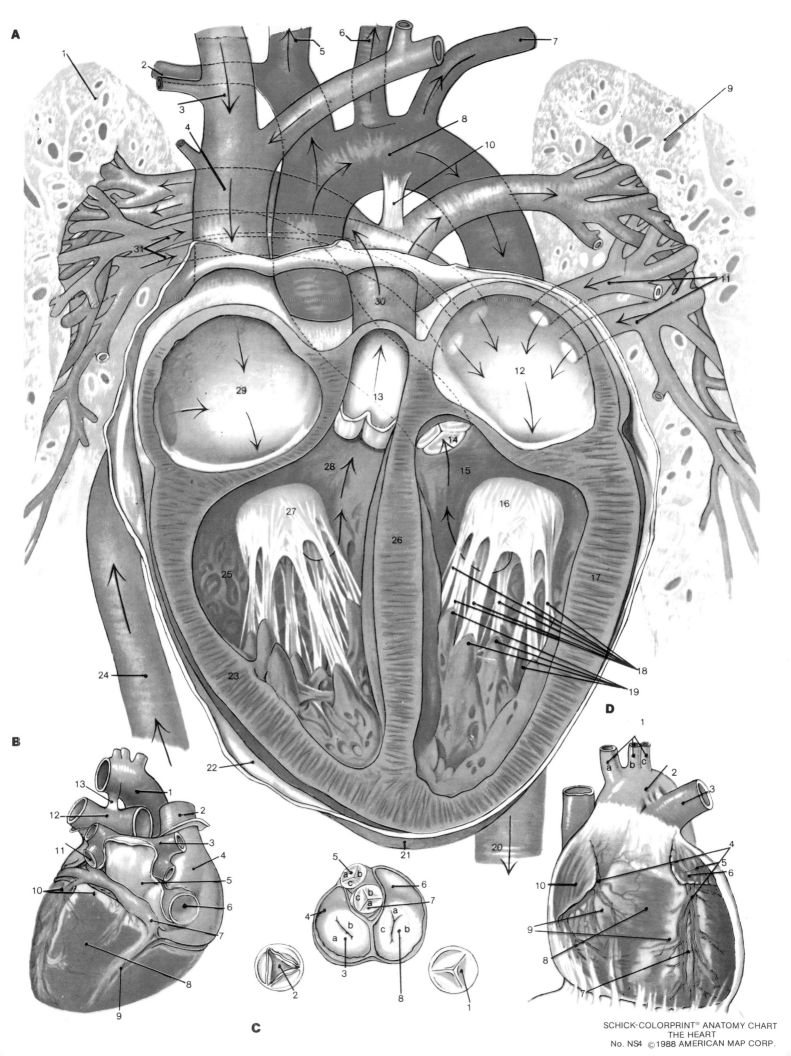

SCHICK-COLORPRINT® ANATOMY CHART
THE HEART
No. NS4 ©1988 AMERICAN MAP CORP.

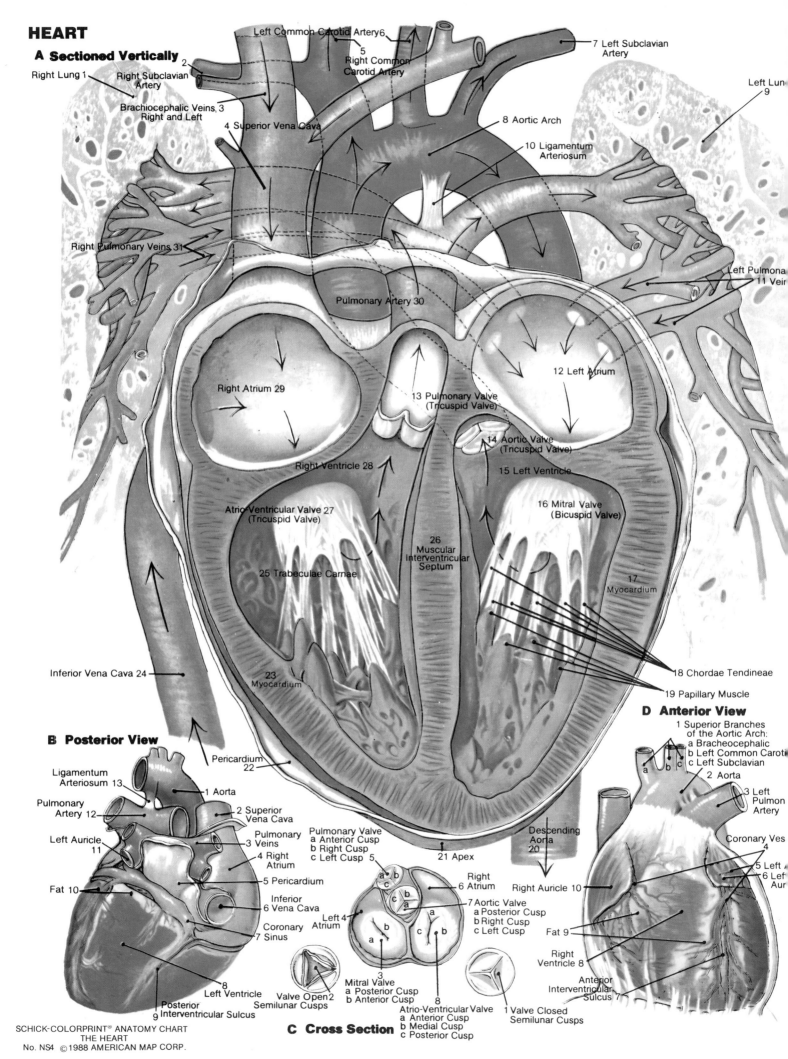

HEART

A Sectioned Vertically

Left Common Carotid Artery 6

5 Right Common Carotid Artery

7 Left Subclavian Artery

2

Right Lung 1

Right Subclavian Artery

Left Lun 9

Brachiocephalic Veins, 3 Right and Left

8 Aortic Arch

4 Superior Vena Cava

10 Ligamentum Arteriosum

Right Pulmonary Veins 31

Left Pulmona 11 Veir

Pulmonary Artery 30

Right Atrium 29

12 Left Atrium

13 Pulmonary Valve (Tricuspid Valve)

14 Aortic Valve (Tricuspid Valve)

Right Ventricle 28

15 Left Ventricle

16 Mitral Valve (Bicuspid Valve)

Atrio-Ventricular Valve 27 (Tricuspid Valve)

17 Myocardium

26 Muscular Interventricular Septum

25 Trabeculae Carnae

18 Chordae Tendineae

Inferior Vena Cava 24

19 Papillary Muscle

23 Myocardium

D Anterior View

1 Superior Branches of the Aortic Arch:
a Bracheocephalic
b Left Common Caroti
c Left Subclavian

B Posterior View

Ligamentum Arteriosum 13

1 Aorta

2 Aorta

Pericardium 22

3 Left Pulmon Artery

Pulmonary Artery 12

2 Superior Vena Cava

Pulmonary 3 Veins

Coronary Ves 4

Left Auricle 11

4 Right Atrium

5 Left
6 Lef Aur

Fat 10

5 Pericardium

Inferior 6 Vena Cava

Descending Aorta 20

Coronary 7 Sinus

Right 6 Atrium

Right Auricle 10

21 Apex

7 Aortic Valve
a Posterior Cusp
b Right Cusp
c Left Cusp

Fat 9

Pulmonary Valve
a Anterior Cusp
b Right Cusp
c Left Cusp 5

Right Ventricle 8

8 Left Ventricle

Posterior 9 Interventricular Sulcus

Valve Open 2 Semilunar Cusps

Left 4 Atrium

Anterior Interventricular Sulcus 7

C Cross Section

Mitral Valve
a Posterior Cusp
b Anterior Cusp 3

Atrio-Ventricular Valve
a Anterior Cusp
b Medial Cusp
c Posterior Cusp 8

1 Valve Closed Semilunar Cusps

SCHICK-COLORPRINT® ANATOMY CHART
THE HEART
No. NS4 © 1988 AMERICAN MAP CORP.

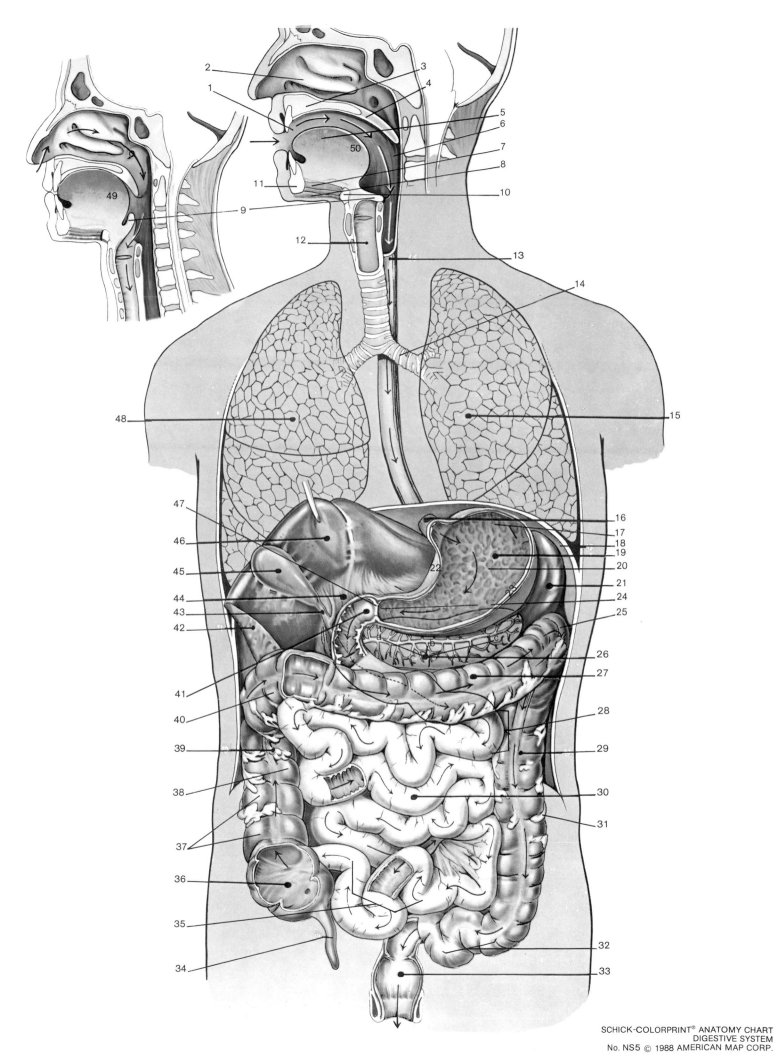

DIGESTIVE SYSTEM

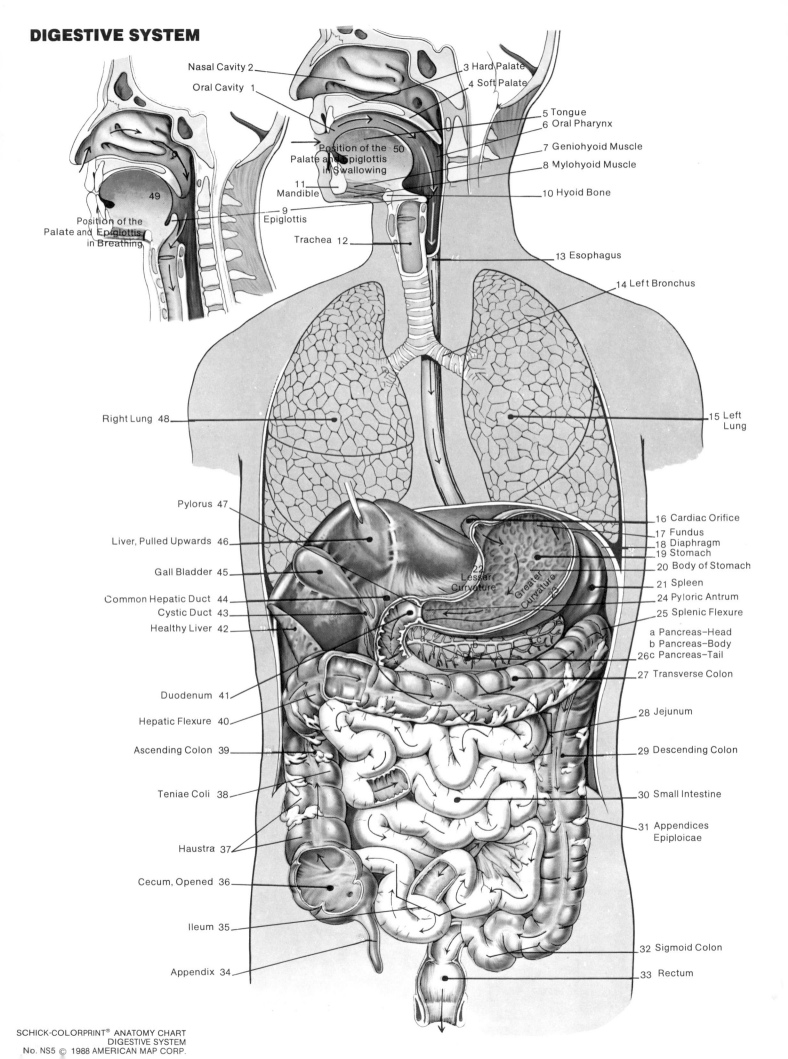

Nasal Cavity 2
Oral Cavity 1
3 Hard Palate
4 Soft Palate
5 Tongue
6 Oral Pharynx
7 Geniohyoid Muscle
8 Mylohyoid Muscle
Position of the 50
Palate and Epiglottis
in Swallowing
11 Mandible
10 Hyoid Bone
9 Epiglottis
Position of the
Palate and Epiglottis
in Breathing
49
Trachea 12
13 Esophagus
14 Left Bronchus
Right Lung 48
15 Left Lung
Pylorus 47
16 Cardiac Orifice
17 Fundus
Liver, Pulled Upwards 46
18 Diaphragm
19 Stomach
20 Body of Stomach
Gall Bladder 45
22 Lesser Curvature
Greater Curvature
21 Spleen
Common Hepatic Duct 44
24 Pyloric Antrum
Cystic Duct 43
25 Splenic Flexure
Healthy Liver 42
a Pancreas–Head
b Pancreas–Body
26c Pancreas–Tail
27 Transverse Colon
Duodenum 41
28 Jejunum
Hepatic Flexure 40
29 Descending Colon
Ascending Colon 39
Teniae Coli 38
30 Small Intestine
31 Appendices Epiploicae
Haustra 37
Cecum, Opened 36
Ileum 35
32 Sigmoid Colon
Appendix 34
33 Rectum

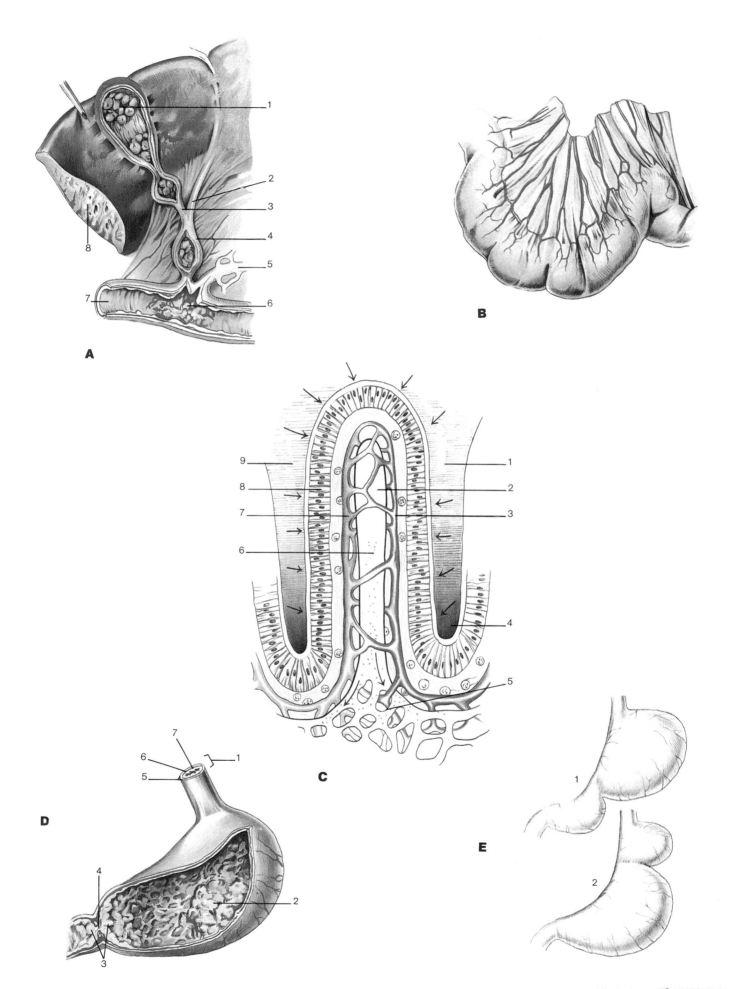

A

B

C

D

E

SCHICK-COLORPRINT® ANATOMY CHART
INTESTINAL VILLUS & DIGESTIVE DISORDERS
No. NS6 © 1988 AMERICAN MAP CORP.

INTESTINAL VILLUS & DIGESTIVE DISORDERS

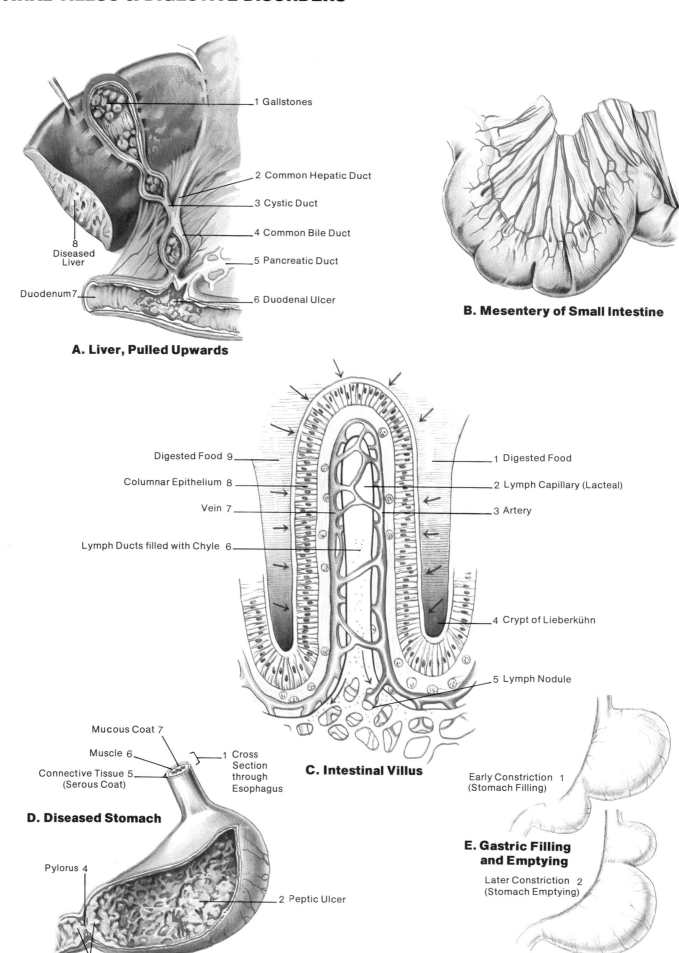

A. Liver, Pulled Upwards

- 1 Gallstones
- 2 Common Hepatic Duct
- 3 Cystic Duct
- 4 Common Bile Duct
- 5 Pancreatic Duct
- 6 Duodenal Ulcer
- 8 Diseased Liver
- Duodenum 7

B. Mesentery of Small Intestine

C. Intestinal Villus

- Digested Food 9
- Columnar Epithelium 8
- Vein 7
- Lymph Ducts filled with Chyle 6
- 1 Digested Food
- 2 Lymph Capillary (Lacteal)
- 3 Artery
- 4 Crypt of Lieberkühn
- 5 Lymph Nodule

D. Diseased Stomach

- Mucous Coat 7
- Muscle 6
- Connective Tissue 5 (Serous Coat)
- 1 Cross Section through Esophagus
- Pylorus 4
- 2 Peptic Ulcer
- 3 Pylorus Deformed by Carcinoma

E. Gastric Filling and Emptying

- Early Constriction 1 (Stomach Filling)
- Later Constriction 2 (Stomach Emptying)

SCHICK-COLORPRINT® ANATOMY CHART
INTESTINAL VILLUS & DIGESTIVE DISORDERS
No. NS6 © 1988 AMERICAN MAP CORP.

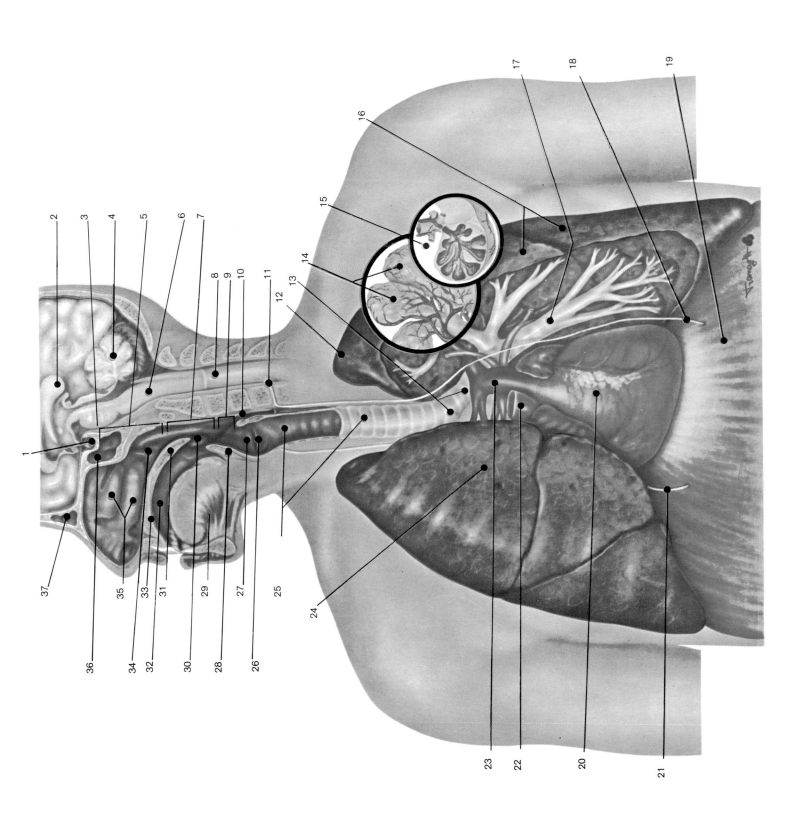

SCHICK-COLORPRINT® ANATOMY CHART
RESPIRATORY TRACT
No. NS7 © 1988 AMERICAN MAP CORP.

RESPIRATORY TRACT

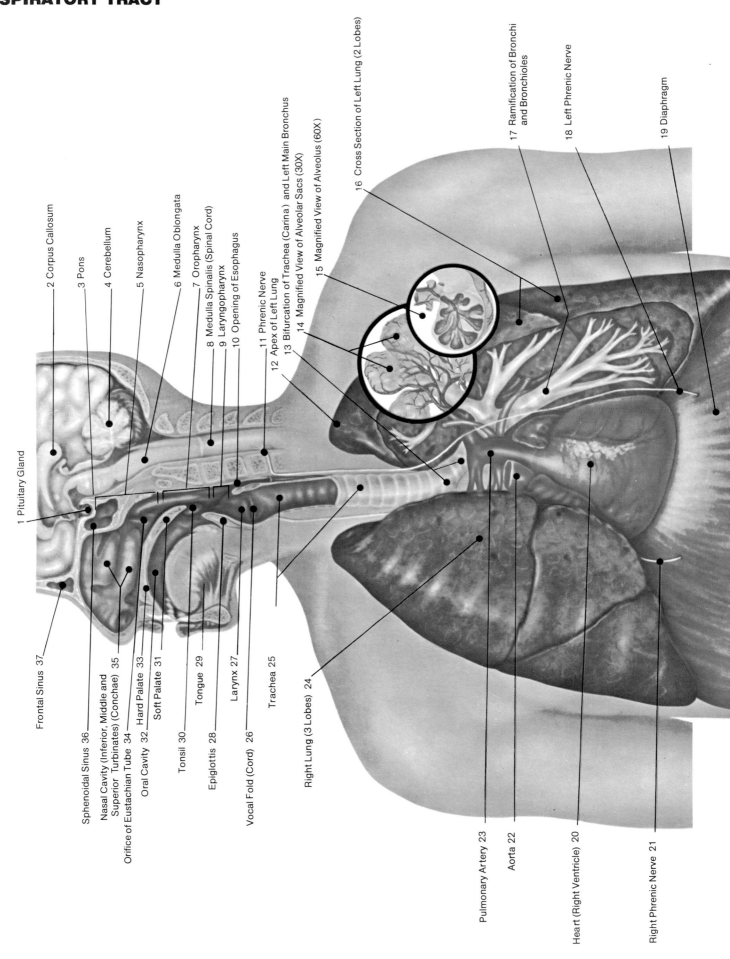

1 Pituitary Gland
2 Corpus Callosum
3 Pons
4 Cerebellum
5 Nasopharynx
6 Medulla Oblongata
7 Oropharynx
8 Medulla Spinalis (Spinal Cord)
9 Laryngopharynx
10 Opening of Esophagus
11 Phrenic Nerve
12 Apex of Left Lung
13 Bifurcation of Trachea (Carina) and Left Main Bronchus
14 Magnified View of Alveolar Sacs (30X)
15 Magnified View of Alveolus (60X)
16 Cross Section of Left Lung (2 Lobes)
17 Ramification of Bronchi and Bronchioles
18 Left Phrenic Nerve
19 Diaphragm

Frontal Sinus 37
Sphenoidal Sinus 36
Nasal Cavity (Inferior, Middle and Superior Turbinates) (Conchae) 35
Orifice of Eustachian Tube 34
Hard Palate 33
Oral Cavity 32
Soft Palate 31
Tonsil 30
Tongue 29
Epiglottis 28
Larynx 27
Vocal Fold (Cord) 26
Trachea 25
Right Lung (3 Lobes) 24

Pulmonary Artery 23
Aorta 22
Heart (Right Ventricle) 20
Right Phrenic Nerve 21

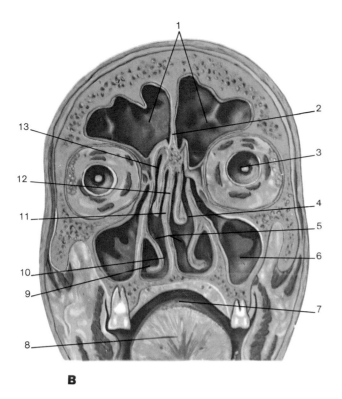

B

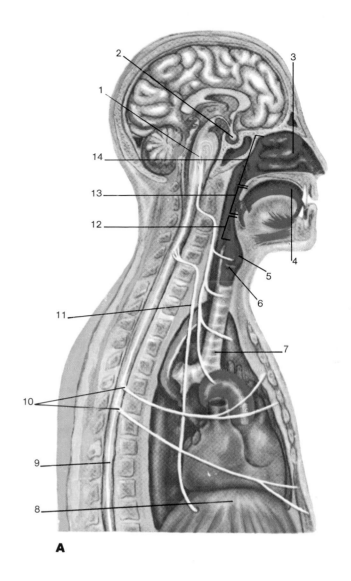

A

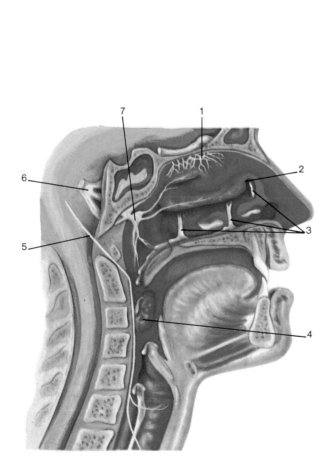

D

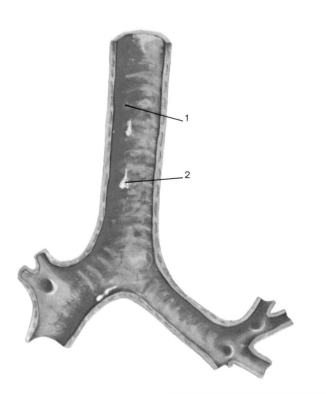

E

SCHICK-COLORPRINT® ANATOMY CHART
NERVOUS CONTROL OF RESPIRATION AND SYMPTOMS OF INFECTION
No. NS8 © 1988 AMERICAN MAP CORP.

NERVOUS CONTROL OF RESPIRATION AND SYMPTOMS OF INFECTIONS

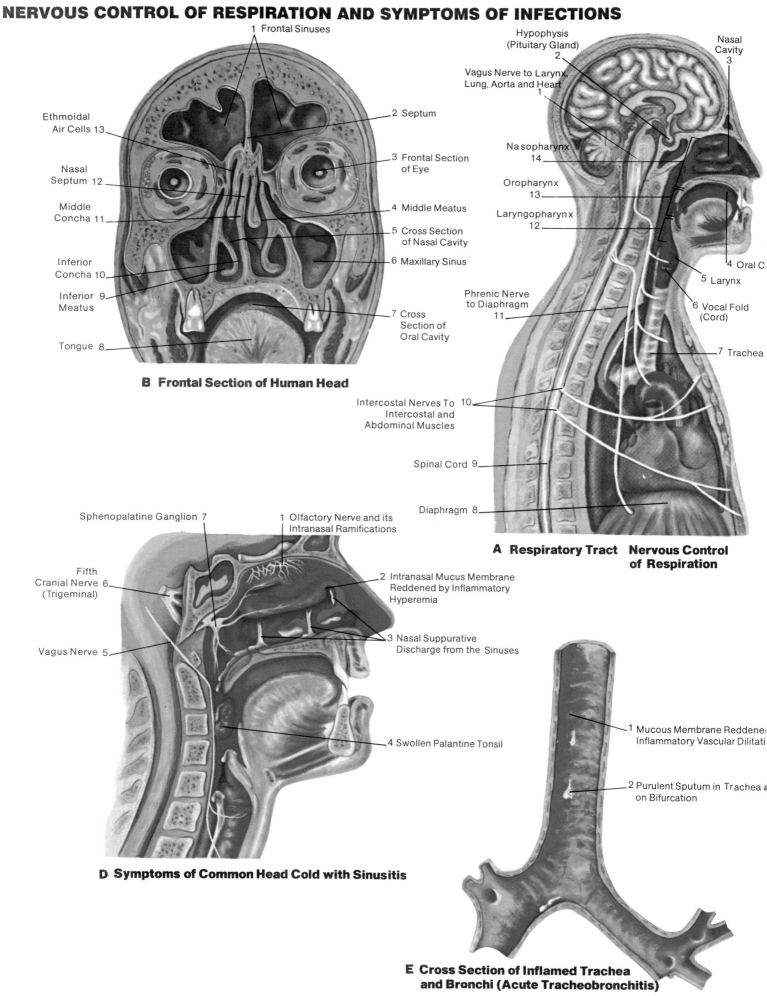

B Frontal Section of Human Head

1 Frontal Sinuses
2 Septum
3 Frontal Section of Eye
4 Middle Meatus
5 Cross Section of Nasal Cavity
6 Maxillary Sinus
7 Cross Section of Oral Cavity
Ethmoidal Air Cells 13
Nasal Septum 12
Middle Concha 11
Inferior Concha 10
Inferior 9 Meatus
Tongue 8

A Respiratory Tract   Nervous Control of Respiration

Hypophysis (Pituitary Gland) 2
Vagus Nerve to Larynx, Lung, Aorta and Heart 1
Nasal Cavity 3
Nasopharynx 14
Oropharynx 13
Laryngopharynx 12
4 Oral C
5 Larynx
6 Vocal Fold (Cord)
7 Trachea
Phrenic Nerve to Diaphragm 11
Intercostal Nerves To 10 Intercostal and Abdominal Muscles
Spinal Cord 9
Diaphragm 8

D Symptoms of Common Head Cold with Sinusitis

Sphenopalatine Ganglion 7
1 Olfactory Nerve and its Intranasal Ramifications
Fifth Cranial Nerve 6 (Trigeminal)
2 Intranasal Mucus Membrane Reddened by Inflammatory Hyperemia
Vagus Nerve 5
3 Nasal Suppurative Discharge from the Sinuses
4 Swollen Palantine Tonsil

E Cross Section of Inflamed Trachea and Bronchi (Acute Tracheobronchitis)

1 Mucous Membrane Reddene Inflammatory Vascular Dilitati
2 Purulent Sputum in Trachea on Bifurcation

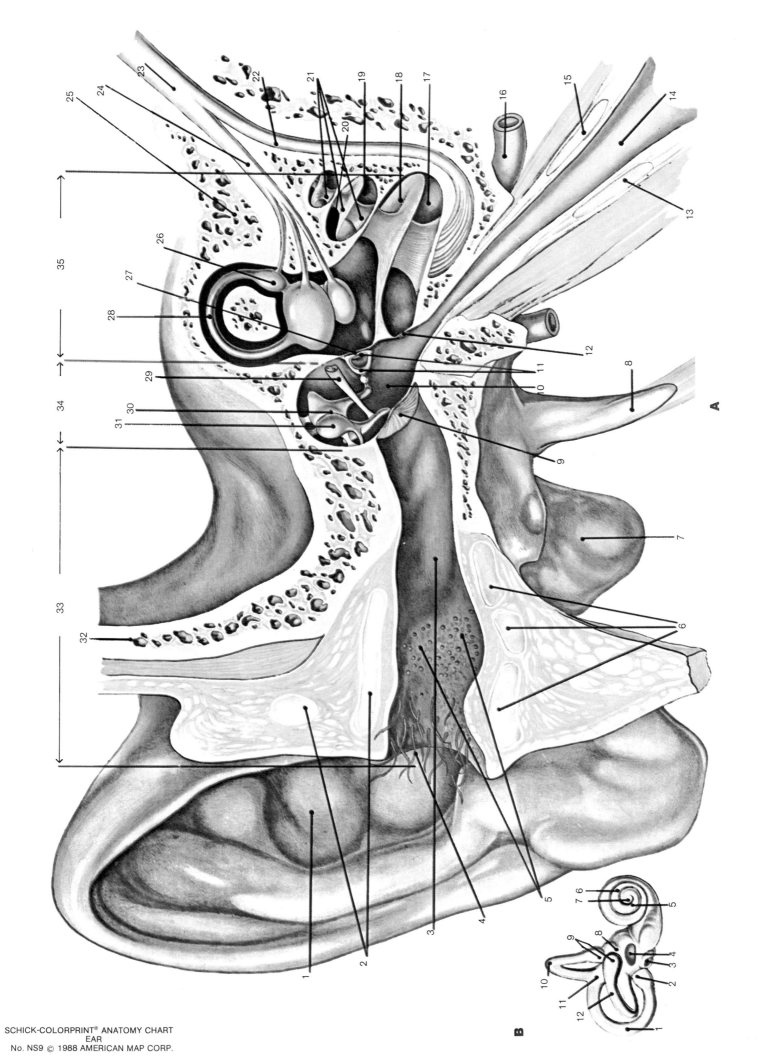

EAR

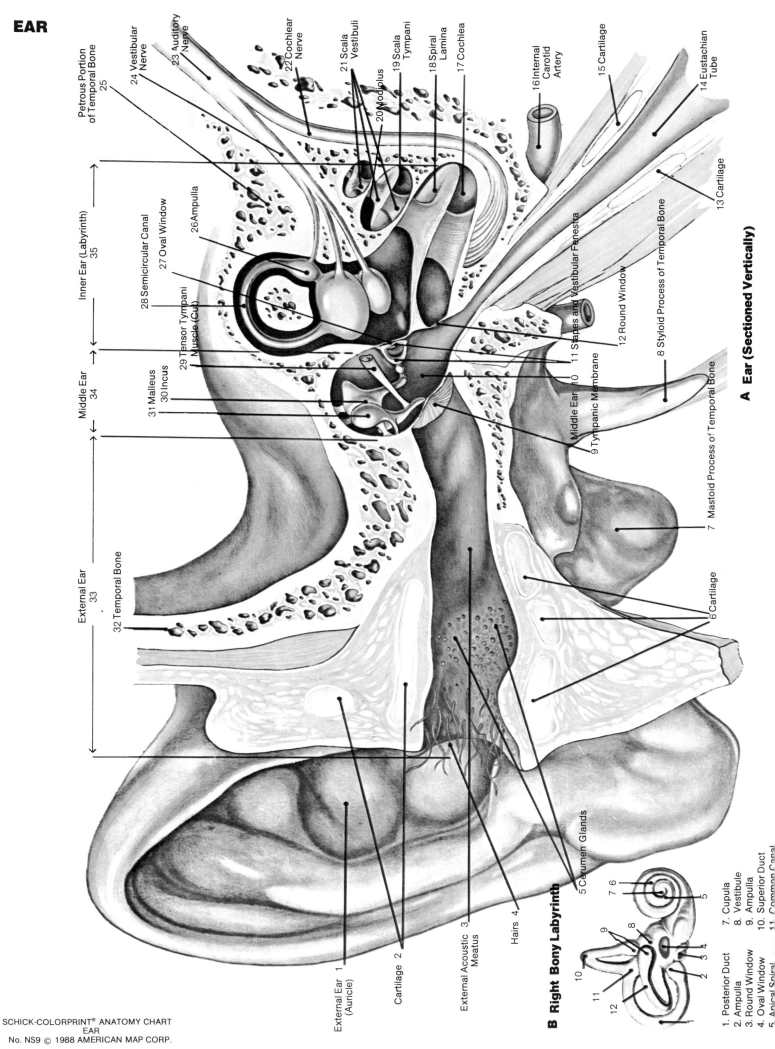

Petrous Portion of Temporal Bone 25

24 Vestibular Nerve

23 Auditory Nerve

22 Cochlear Nerve

21 Scala Vestibuli

20 Modiolus

19 Scala Tympani

18 Spiral Lamina

17 Cochlea

16 Internal Carotid Artery

15 Cartilage

14 Eustachian Tube

13 Cartilage

Inner Ear (Labyrinth) 35

26 Ampulla

27 Oval Window

28 Semicircular Canal

29 Tensor Tympani Muscle (Cut)

11 Stapes and Vestibular Fenestra

12 Round Window

8 Styloid Process of Temporal Bone

Middle Ear 34

31 Malleus

30 Incus

Middle Ear 10

9 Tympanic Membrane

7 Mastoid Process of Temporal Bone

External Ear 33

32 Temporal Bone

6 Cartilage

External Ear 1 (Auricle)

Cartilage 2

External Acoustic Meatus

Hairs 4

3 External Spiral

5 Cerumen Glands

A Ear (Sectioned Vertically)

B Right Bony Labyrinth

7 6

9

8

5

10

4

11

3

2

12

1

1. Posterior Duct
2. Ampulla
3. Round Window
4. Oval Window
5. Apical Spiral
6.
7. Cupula
8. Vestibule
9. Ampulla
10. Superior Duct
11. Common Canal

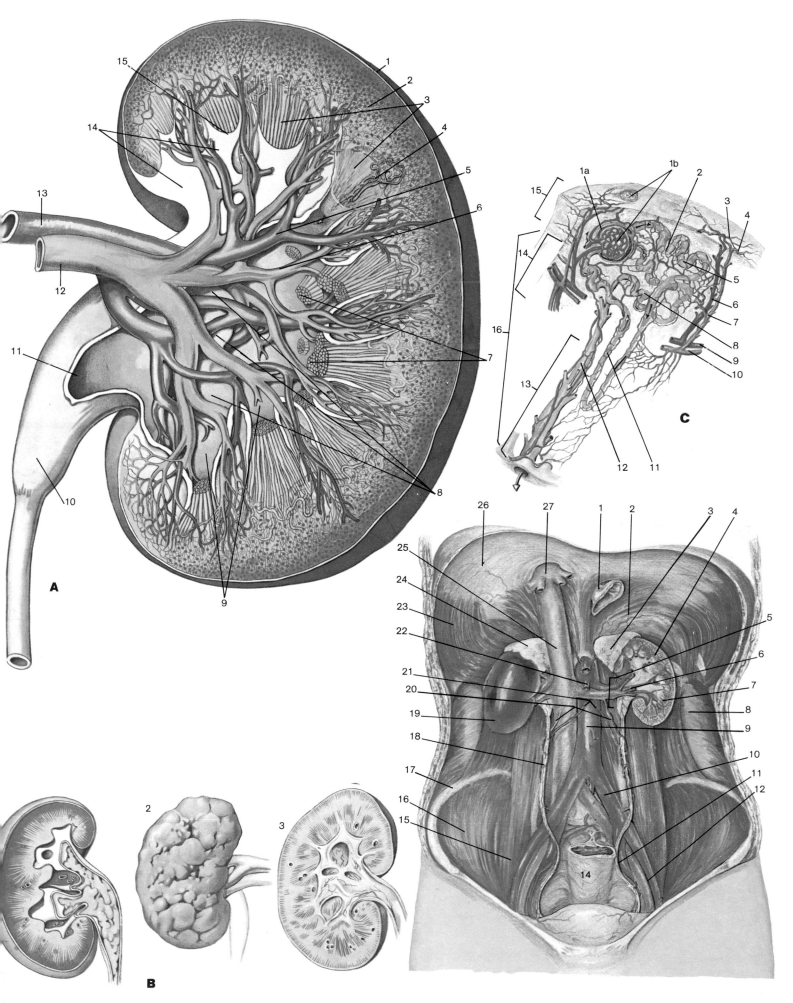

SCHICK-COLORPRINT® ANATOMY CHART
KIDNEYS
No. NS10 © 1988 AMERICAN MAP CORP.

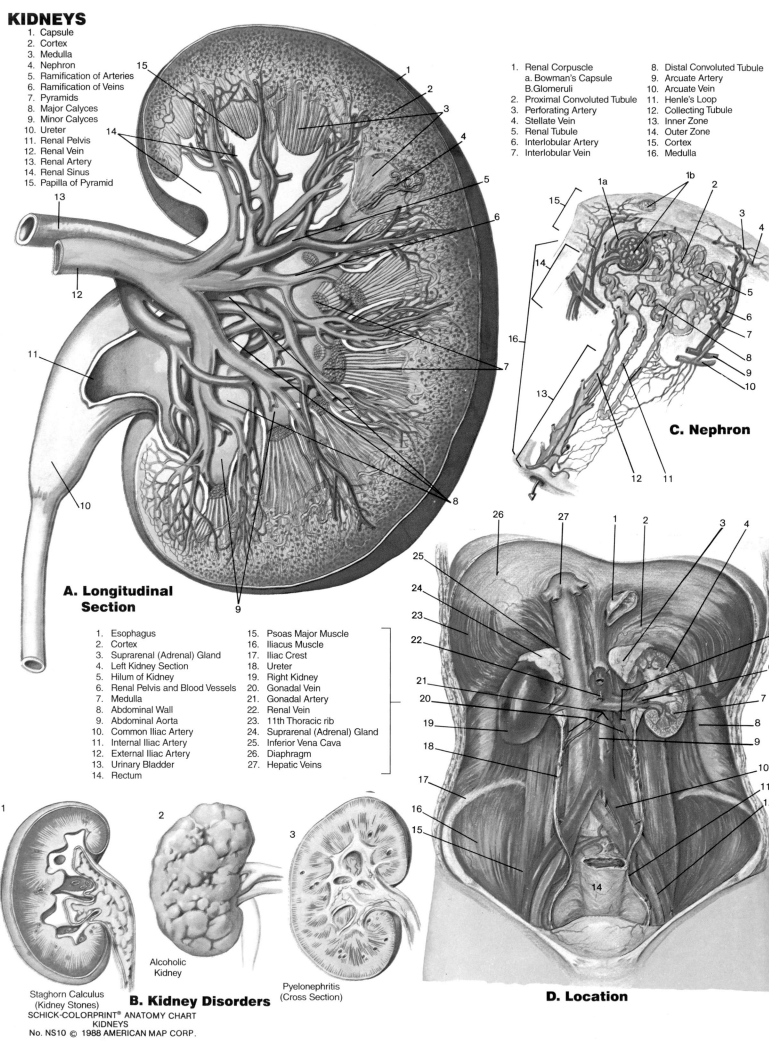

KIDNEYS

1. Capsule
2. Cortex
3. Medulla
4. Nephron
5. Ramification of Arteries
6. Ramification of Veins
7. Pyramids
8. Major Calyces
9. Minor Calyces
10. Ureter
11. Renal Pelvis
12. Renal Vein
13. Renal Artery
14. Renal Sinus
15. Papilla of Pyramid

A. Longitudinal Section

1. Renal Corpuscle
   a. Bowman's Capsule
   B. Glomeruli
2. Proximal Convoluted Tubule
3. Perforating Artery
4. Stellate Vein
5. Renal Tubule
6. Interlobular Artery
7. Interlobular Vein
8. Distal Convoluted Tubule
9. Arcuate Artery
10. Arcuate Vein
11. Henle's Loop
12. Collecting Tubule
13. Inner Zone
14. Outer Zone
15. Cortex
16. Medulla

C. Nephron

1. Esophagus
2. Cortex
3. Suprarenal (Adrenal) Gland
4. Left Kidney Section
5. Hilum of Kidney
6. Renal Pelvis and Blood Vessels
7. Medulla
8. Abdominal Wall
9. Abdominal Aorta
10. Common Iliac Artery
11. Internal Iliac Artery
12. External Iliac Artery
13. Urinary Bladder
14. Rectum
15. Psoas Major Muscle
16. Iliacus Muscle
17. Iliac Crest
18. Ureter
19. Right Kidney
20. Gonadal Vein
21. Gonadal Artery
22. Renal Vein
23. 11th Thoracic rib
24. Suprarenal (Adrenal) Gland
25. Inferior Vena Cava
26. Diaphragm
27. Hepatic Veins

Staghorn Calculus
(Kidney Stones)

Alcoholic
Kidney

Pyelonephritis
(Cross Section)

B. Kidney Disorders

D. Location

SCHICK-COLORPRINT® ANATOMY CHART
KIDNEYS
No. NS10 © 1988 AMERICAN MAP CORP.

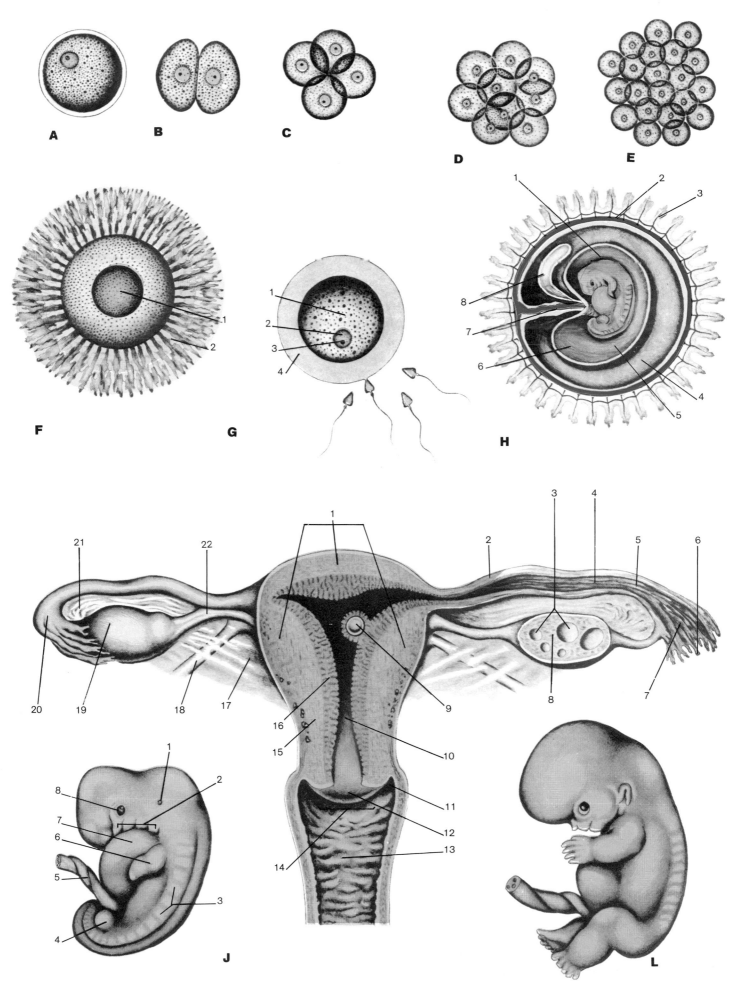

DEVELOPMENT OF THE HUMAN EMBRYO

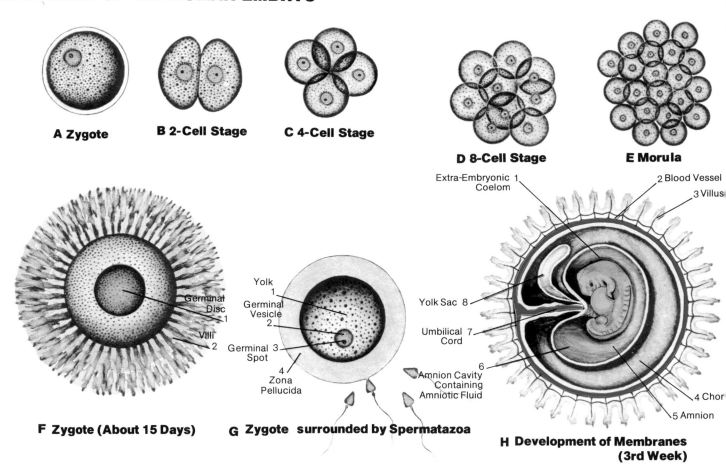

A Zygote

B 2-Cell Stage

C 4-Cell Stage

D 8-Cell Stage

E Morula

Extra-Embryonic 1
Coelom

2 Blood Vessel

3 Villus

Germinal
Disc
1

Villi
2

Yolk
1
Germinal
Vesicle
2

Germinal 3
Spot

4
Zona
Pellucida

Yolk Sac 8

Umbilical 7
Cord

6

Amnion Cavity
Containing
Amniotic Fluid

4 Chor

5 Amnion

F Zygote (About 15 Days)

G Zygote surrounded by Spermatazoa

H Development of Membranes (3rd Week)

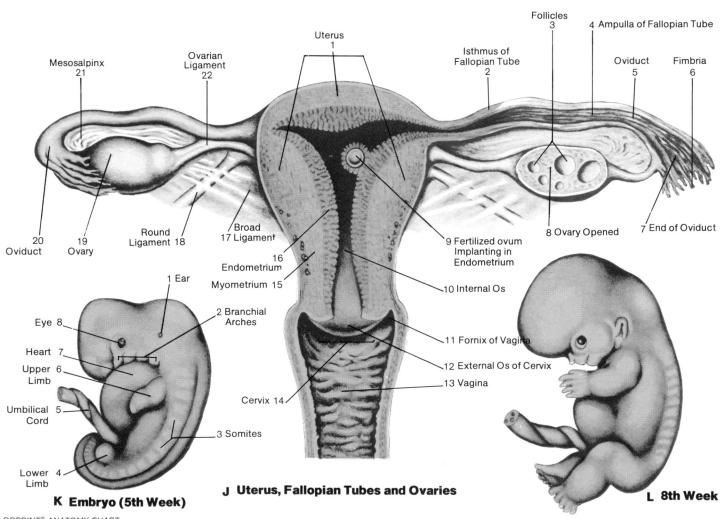

Mesosalpinx
21

Ovarian
Ligament
22

Uterus
1

Isthmus of
Fallopian Tube
2

Follicles
3

4 Ampulla of Fallopian Tube

Oviduct
5

Fimbria
6

20
Oviduct

19
Ovary

Round
Ligament 18

Broad
17 Ligament

16

Endometrium

Myometrium 15

9 Fertilized ovum
Implanting in
Endometrium

10 Internal Os

8 Ovary Opened

7 End of Oviduct

1 Ear

2 Branchial
Arches

Eye 8

Heart 7

Upper 6
Limb

Umbilical 5
Cord

Lower 4
Limb

3 Somites

11 Fornix of Vagina

12 External Os of Cervix

13 Vagina

Cervix 14

K Embryo (5th Week)

J Uterus, Fallopian Tubes and Ovaries

L 8th Week

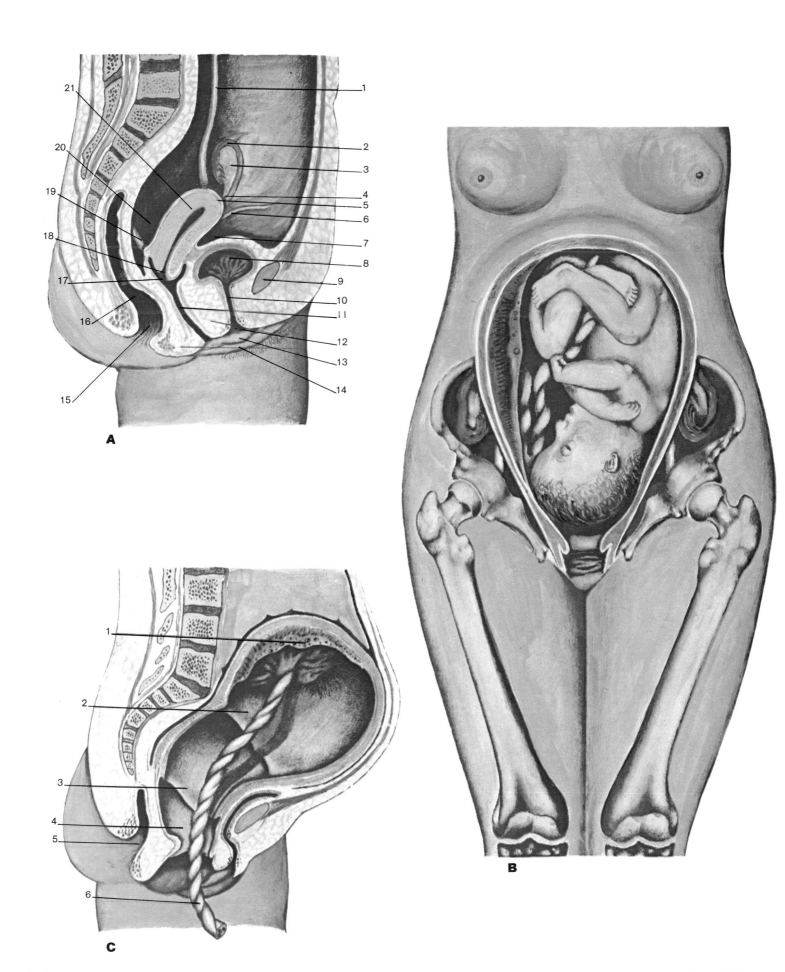

A

21
20
19
18
17
16
15

1
2
3
4
5
6
7
8
9
10
11
12
13
14

B

C

1
2
3
4
5
6

FEMALE REPRODUCTIVE ORGANS AND PREGNANCY AT TERM

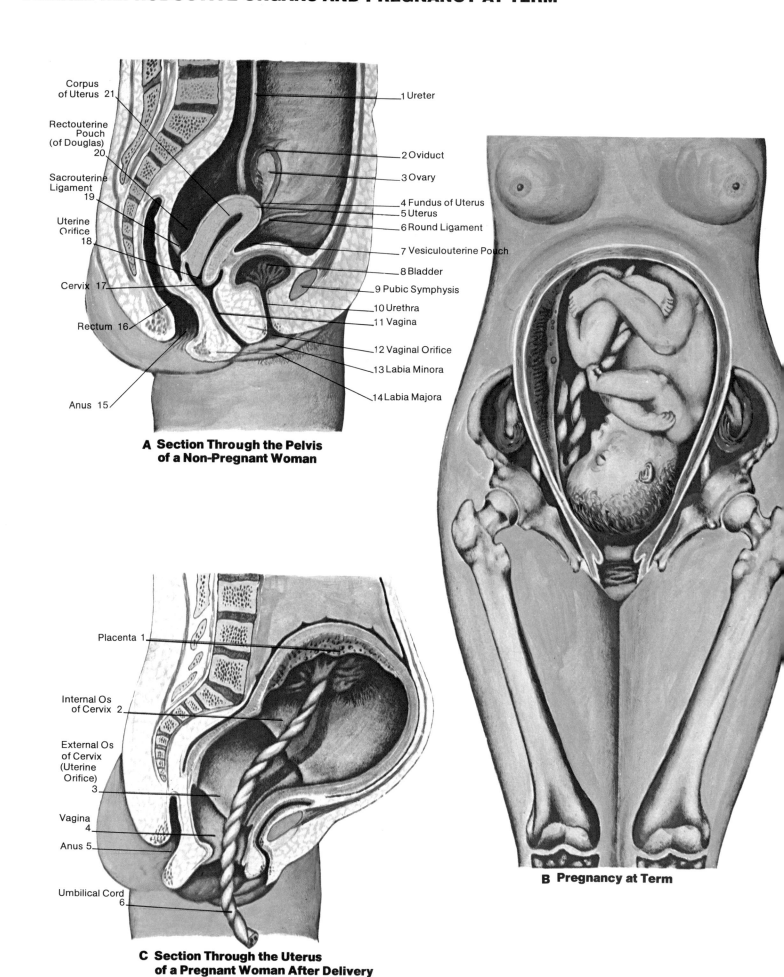

Corpus of Uterus 21
Rectouterine Pouch (of Douglas) 20
Sacrouterine Ligament 19
Uterine Orifice 18
Cervix 17
Rectum 16
Anus 15

1 Ureter
2 Oviduct
3 Ovary
4 Fundus of Uterus
5 Uterus
6 Round Ligament
7 Vesiculouterine Pouch
8 Bladder
9 Pubic Symphysis
10 Urethra
11 Vagina
12 Vaginal Orifice
13 Labia Minora
14 Labia Majora

A Section Through the Pelvis of a Non-Pregnant Woman

Placenta 1
Internal Os of Cervix 2
External Os of Cervix (Uterine Orifice) 3
Vagina 4
Anus 5
Umbilical Cord 6

C Section Through the Uterus of a Pregnant Woman After Delivery

B Pregnancy at Term

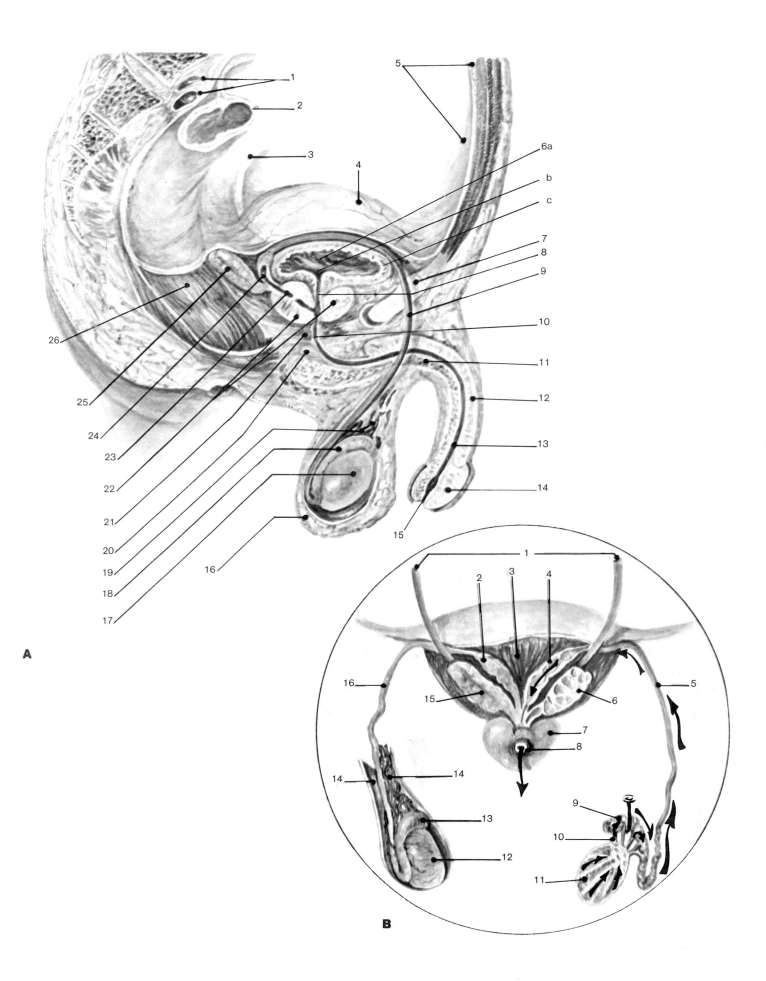

A

B

MALE REPRODUCTIVE ORGANS

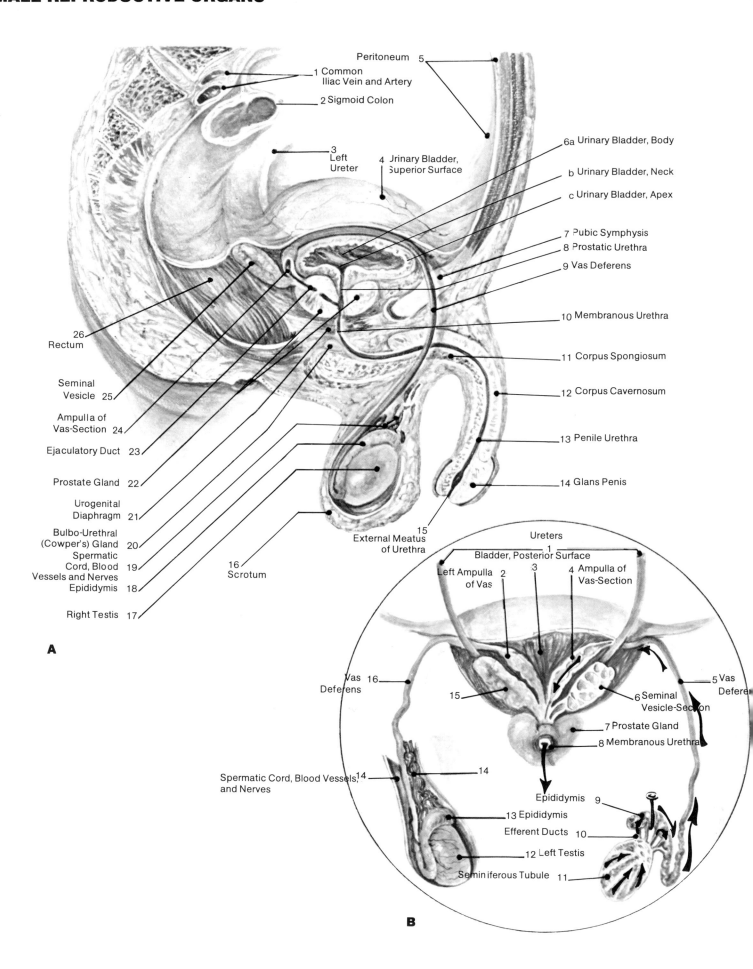

Peritoneum 5

1 Common
  Iliac Vein and Artery

2 Sigmoid Colon

3 Left Ureter

4 Urinary Bladder, Superior Surface

6a Urinary Bladder, Body

b Urinary Bladder, Neck

c Urinary Bladder, Apex

7 Pubic Symphysis
8 Prostatic Urethra
9 Vas Deferens

10 Membranous Urethra

11 Corpus Spongiosum

12 Corpus Cavernosum

13 Penile Urethra

14 Glans Penis

15 External Meatus of Urethra

16 Scrotum

26 Rectum

Seminal Vesicle 25

Ampulla of Vas-Section 24

Ejaculatory Duct 23

Prostate Gland 22

Urogenital Diaphragm 21

Bulbo-Urethral (Cowper's) Gland 20

Spermatic Cord, Blood Vessels and Nerves 19

Epididymis 18

Right Testis 17

A

Ureters

Bladder, Posterior Surface 1

Left Ampulla of Vas 2

3

4 Ampulla of Vas-Section

Vas Deferens 16

15

5 Vas Deferens

6 Seminal Vesicle-Section

7 Prostate Gland

8 Membranous Urethra

Spermatic Cord, Blood Vessels, and Nerves 14

14

Epididymis 9

13 Epididymis

Efferent Ducts 10

12 Left Testis

Seminiferous Tubule 11

B

SCHICK-COLORPRINT® ANATOMY CHART
MALE REPRO. ORGANS
No. NS13 © 1988 AMERICAN MAP CORP.

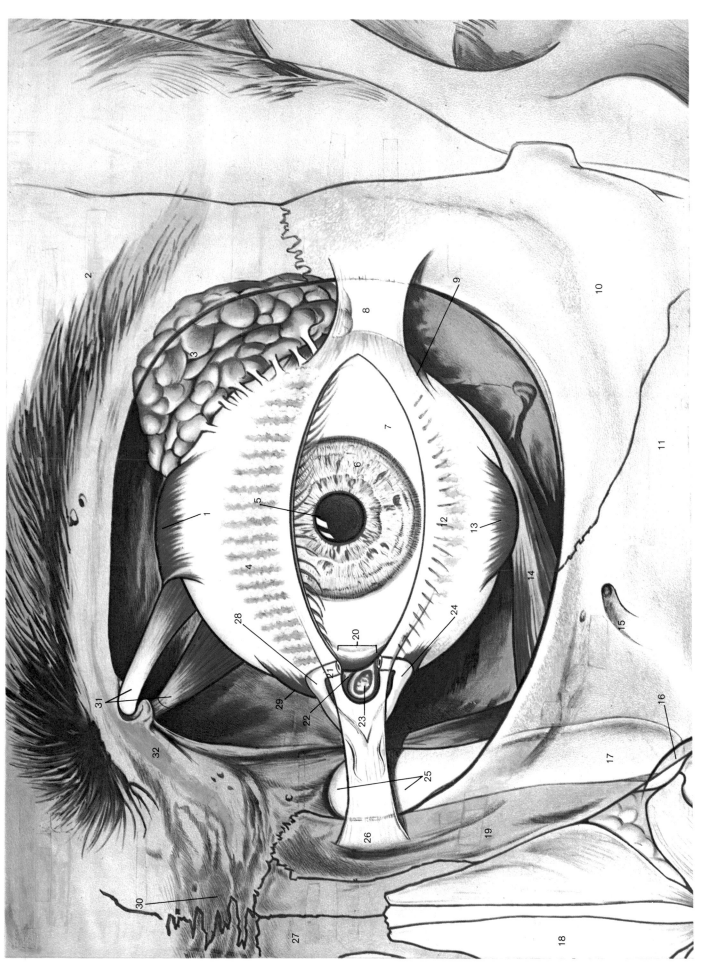

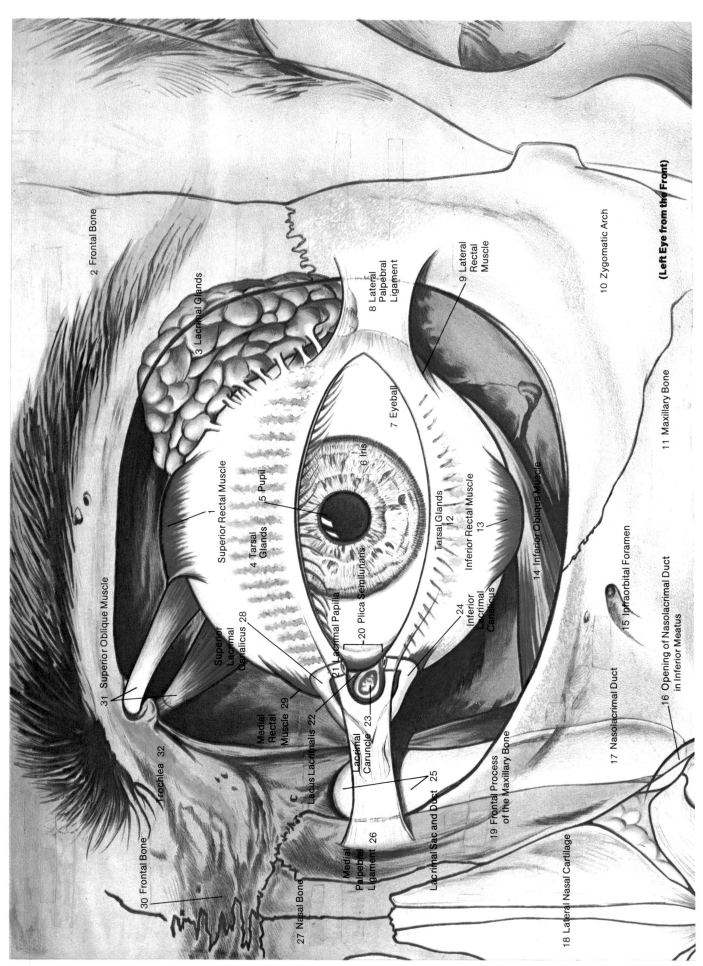

(Left Eye from the Front)

1 Superior Rectal Muscle
2 Frontal Bone
3 Lacrimal Glands
4 Tarsal Glands
5 Pupil
6 Iris
7 Eyeball
8 Lateral Palpebral Ligament
9 Lateral Rectal Muscle
10 Zygomatic Arch
11 Maxillary Bone
12 Tarsal Glands
13 Inferior Rectal Muscle
14 Inferior Oblique Muscle
15 Infraorbital Foramen
16 Opening of Nasolacrimal Duct in Inferior Meatus
17 Nasolacrimal Duct
18 Lateral Nasal Cartilage
19 Frontal Process of the Maxillary Bone
20 Plica Semilunaris
21 Lacrimal Papilla
22 Lacus Lacrimalis
23 Lacrimal Caruncle
24 Inferior Lacrimal Canaliculus
25 Lacrimal Sac and Duct
26 Medial Palpebral Ligament
27 Nasal Bone
28 Superior Lacrimal Canaliculus
29 Medial Rectal Muscle
30 Frontal Bone
31 Superior Oblique Muscle
32 Trochlea

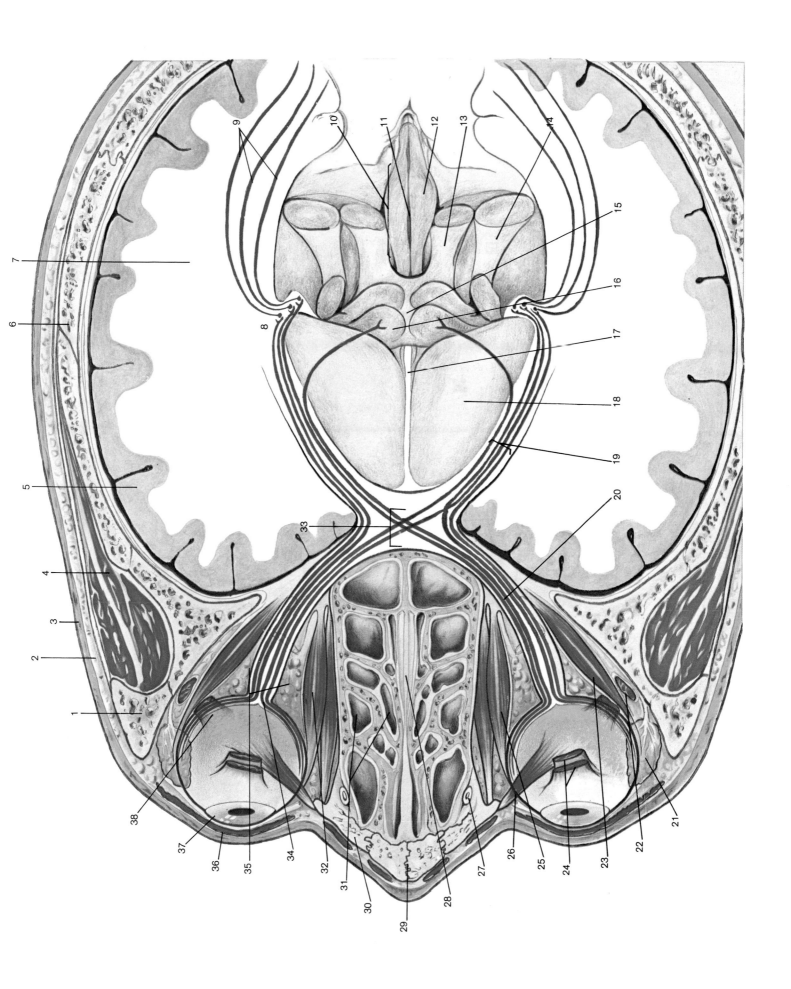

EYE - Sight as a Function of the Brain

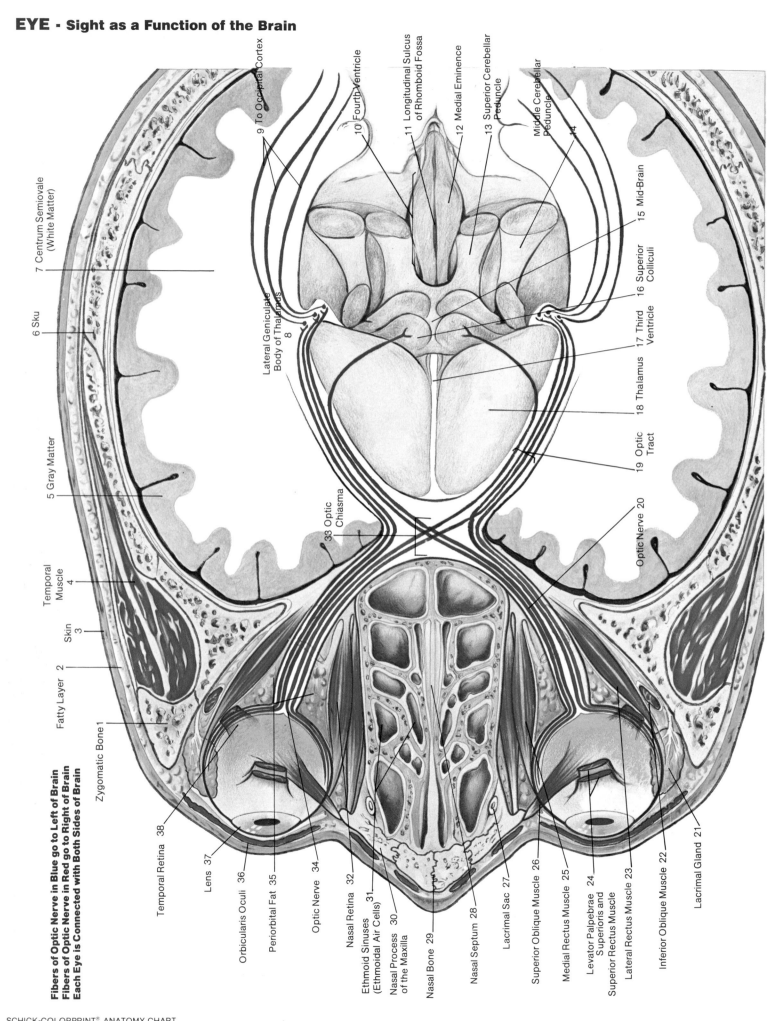

Fibers of Optic Nerve in Blue go to Left of Brain
Fibers of Optic Nerve in Red go to Right of Brain
Each Eye is Connected with Both Sides of Brain

9 To Occipital Cortex
10 Fourth Ventricle
11 Longitudinal Sulcus of Rhomboid Fossa
12 Medial Eminence
13 Superior Cerebellar Peduncle
Middle Cerebellar Peduncle
14
15 Mid-Brain
16 Superior Colliculi
17 Third Ventricle
18 Thalamus
19 Optic Tract
Optic Nerve 20

7 Centrum Semiovale (White Matter)
6 Sku
Lateral Geniculate Body of Thalamus
8
5 Gray Matter
Temporal Muscle 4
Skin 3
Fatty Layer 2
Zygomatic Bone 1
33 Optic Chiasma

Temporal Retina 38
Lens 37
Orbicularis Oculi 36
Periorbital Fat 35
Optic Nerve 34
Nasal Retina 32
Ethmoid Sinuses (Ethmoidal Air Cells) 31
Nasal Process of the Maxilla 30
Nasal Bone 29
Nasal Septum 28
Lacrimal Sac 27
Superior Oblique Muscle 26
Medial Rectus Muscle 25
Levator Palpebrae Superioris and Superior Rectus Muscle 24
Lateral Rectus Muscle 23
Inferior Oblique Muscle 22
Lacrimal Gland 21

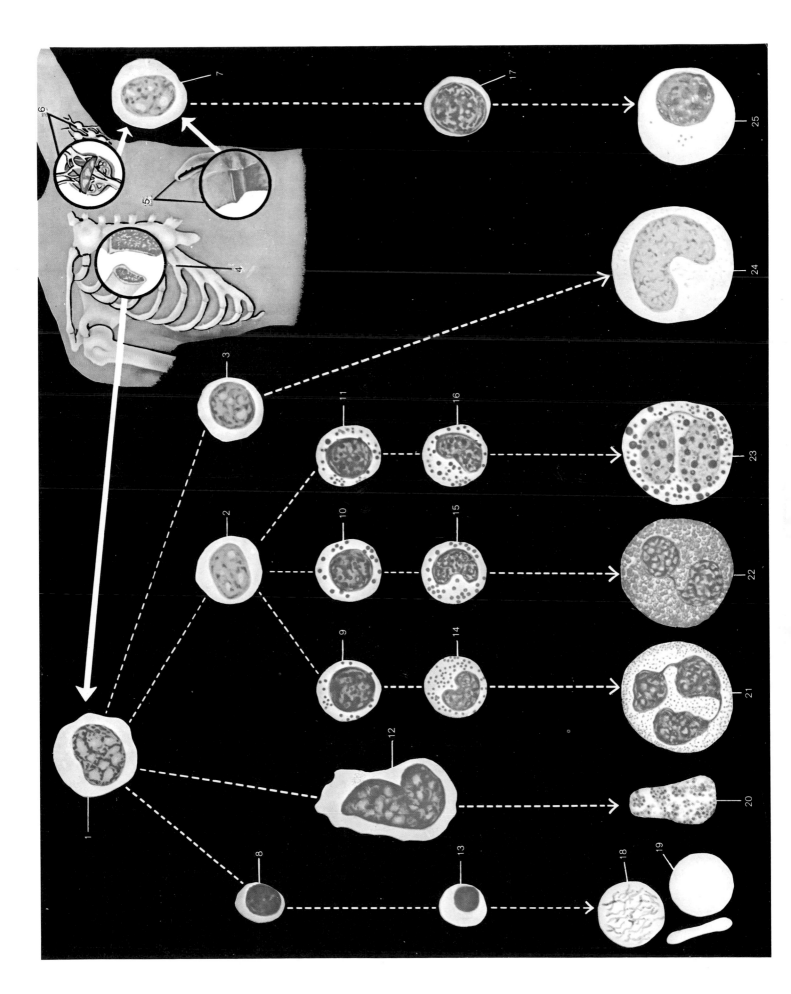

SCHICK-COLORPRINT® ANATOMY CHART
DEVELOPMENT OF BLOOD CELLS
No. NS16 ©1988 AMERICAN MAP CORP.

DEVELOPMENT OF THE BLOOD CELLS

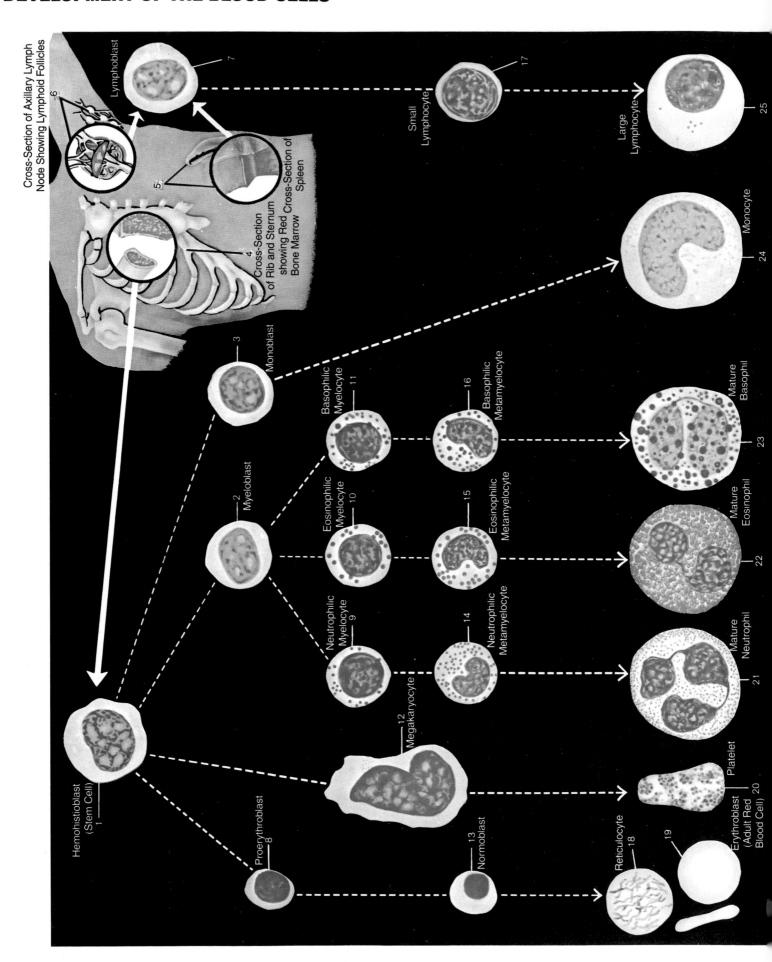

Cross-Section of Axillary Lymph Node Showing Lymphoid Follicles

Lymphoblast 7

Small Lymphocyte 17

Large Lymphocyte 25

6

5

Cross-Section of Rib and Sternum showing Red Bone Marrow 4

Cross-Section of Spleen

Monocyte 24

Monoblast 3

Basophilic Myelocyte 11

Basophilic Metamyelocyte 16

Mature Basophil 23

Myeloblast 2

Eosinophilic Myelocyte 10

Eosinophilic Metamyelocyte 15

Mature Eosinophil 22

Neutrophilic Myelocyte 9

Neutrophilic Metamyelocyte 14

Mature Neutrophil 21

Megakaryocyte 12

Platelet 20

Hemohistoblast (Stem Cell) 1

Proerythroblast 8

Normoblast 13

Reticulocyte 18

Erythroblast (Adult Red Blood Cell) 19

SCHICK-COLORPRINT® ANATOMY CHART
DEVELOPMENT OF BLOOD CELLS
No. NS16 ©1988 AMERICAN MAP CORP.

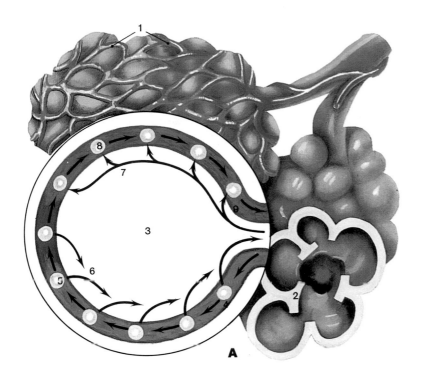

A

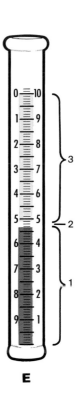

E

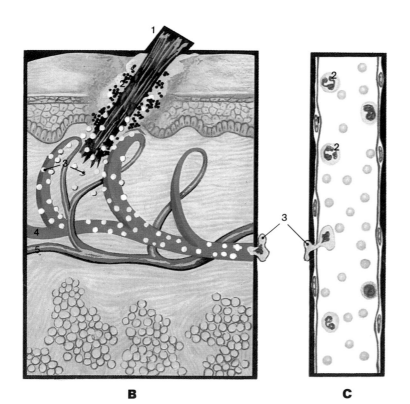

B

C

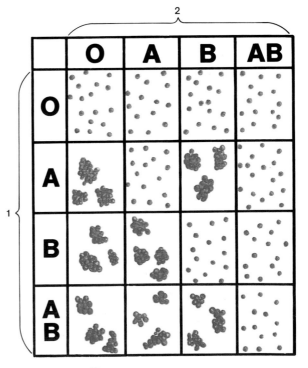

D

BLOOD CELLS

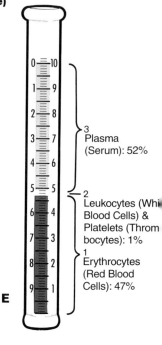

A. Function of the Red Blood Cells

1 Alveolus and Capillary Network
2 Cross-Section of Alveolus Sac
3 Schematic Representation, showing Exchange of Oxygen and Carbon Dioxide
4 Deoxygenated Blood moving through a Capillary
5 Carbon dioxide is released from Red Blood Cells
6 Carbon Dioxide passes into the Alveoli and is expired
7 Oxygen of the inspired air passes through the Alveolar Wall
8 Oxygen enters the Red Blood Cells and is carried to all Organs
9 Alveolar Capillary

E. Normal Blood Cell Volume
(Hematocrit Tube)

3 Plasma (Serum): 52%
2 Leukocytes (White Blood Cells) & Platelets (Thrombocytes): 1%
1 Erythrocytes (Red Blood Cells): 47%

Normal Blood Counts

Erythrocytes (Red Cells): 4,500,000 - 5,000,000/cu.mm.blood
Thrombocytes (Platelets 200,000 - 400,000/cu.mm.blood
Leucocytes (White Cells): 5,000 - 10,000/cu.mm.blood

Neutrophils:	55 - 60%
Lymphocytes:	30 - 35%
Monocytes:	4 - 8%
Eosinophils:	2 - 5%
Basophils:	0 - 1.5%

Hemoglobin
Men: 14.5 - 16.5 gm/100ml blood
Women: 12.7 - 14.7gm/100ml blood

B. Function of the White Blood Cells
(Schematic Cross-Section of Skin)

1 Foreign Body
2 Bacteria on Foreign Body
3 White Cells moving toward Bacteria
4 Arterial Capillary
5 Venous Capillary

C. Microscopic Section of Inflamed Capillary Blood Vessel

1 Endothelial Cell
2 Leukocyte
3 Migration of Leukocyte Through the Capillary Wall

D. Compatibility of Blood Groups
(Large Red Clumps mean Incompatablilty)

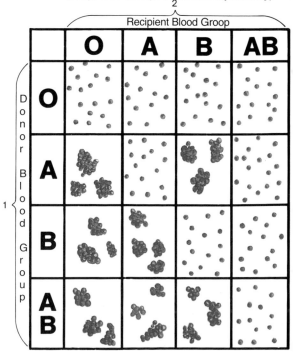

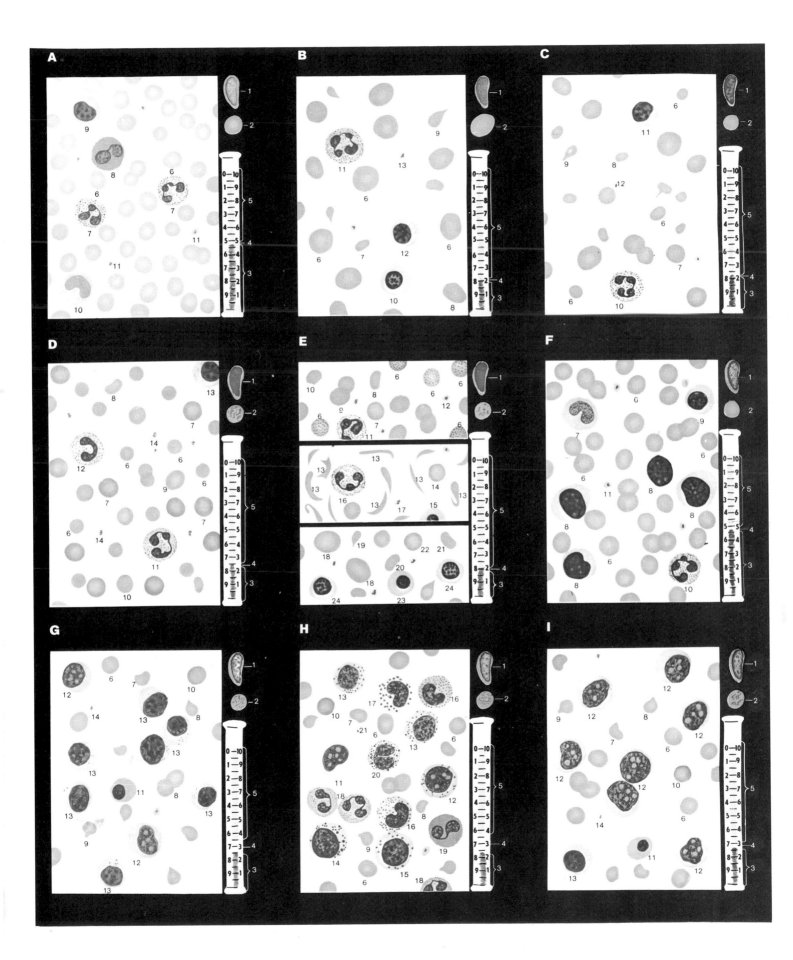

DISEASES OF THE BLOOD CELLS

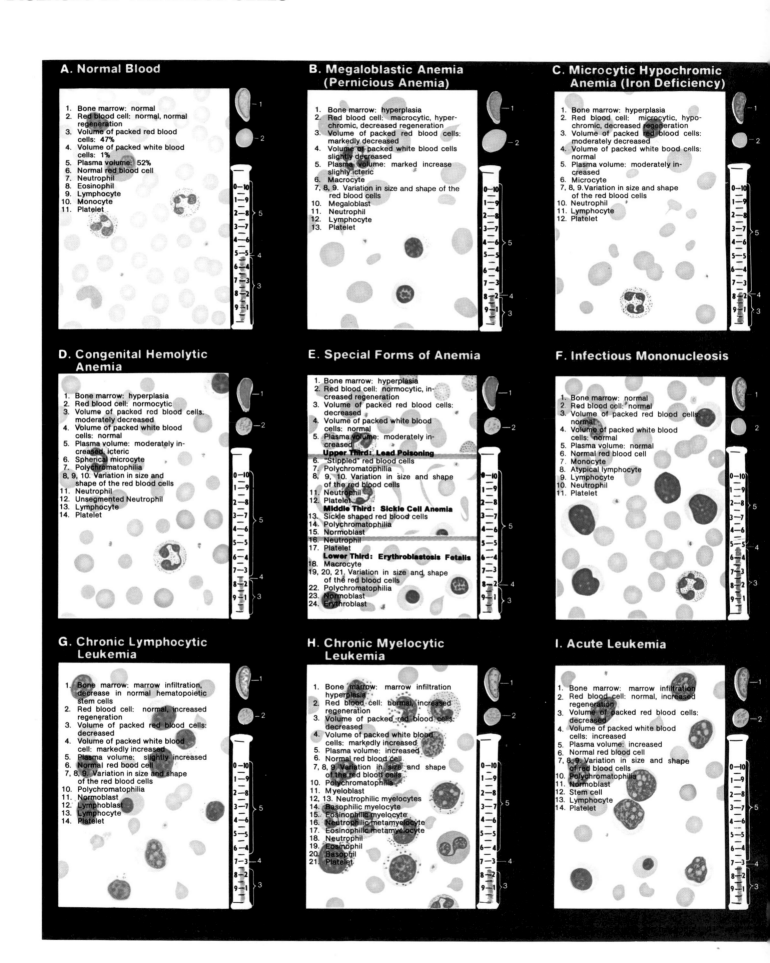

A. Normal Blood

1. Bone marrow: normal
2. Red blood cell: normal, normal regeneration
3. Volume of packed red blood cells: 47%
4. Volume of packed white blood cells: 1%
5. Plasma volume: 52%
6. Normal red blood cell
7. Neutrophil
8. Eosinophil
9. Lymphocyte
10. Monocyte
11. Platelet

B. Megaloblastic Anemia (Pernicious Anemia)

1. Bone marrow: hyperplasia
2. Red blood cell: macrocytic, hyperchromic, decreased regeneration
3. Volume of packed red blood cells: markedly decreased
4. Volume of packed white blood cells slightly decreased
5. Plasma volume: marked increase slighly icteric
6. Macrocyte
7, 8, 9. Variation in size and shape of the red blood cells
10. Megaloblast
11. Neutrophil
12. Lymphocyte
13. Platelet

C. Microcytic Hypochromic Anemia (Iron Deficiency)

1. Bone marrow: hyperplasia
2. Red blood cell: microcytic, hypochromic, decreased regeneration
3. Volume of packed red blood cells: moderately decreased
4. Volume of packed white bood cells: normal
5. Plasma volume: moderately increased
6. Microcyte
7, 8, 9. Variation in size and shape of the red blood cells
10. Neutrophil
11. Lymphocyte
12. Platelet

D. Congenital Hemolytic Anemia

1. Bone marrow: hyperplasia
2. Red blood cell: normocytic
3. Volume of packed red blood cells: moderately decreased
4. Volume of packed white blood cells: normal
5. Plasma volume: moderately increased, icteric
6. Spherical microcyte
7. Polychromatophilia
8, 9, 10. Variation in size and shape of the red blood cells
11. Neutrophil
12. Unsegmented Neutrophil
13. Lymphocyte
14. Platelet

E. Special Forms of Anemia

1. Bone marrow: hyperplasia
2. Red blood cell: normocytic, increased regeneration
3. Volume of packed red blood cells: decreased
4. Volume of packed white blood cells: normal
5. Plasma volume: moderately increased

Upper Third: Lead Poisoning
6. "Stippled" red blood cells
7. Polychromatophilia
8, 9, 10. Variation in size and shape of the red blood cells
11. Neutrophil
12. Platelet

Middle Third: Sickle Cell Anemia
13. Sickle shaped red blood cells
14. Polychromatophilia
15. Normoblast
16. Neutrophil
17. Platelet

Lower Third: Erythroblastosis Fetalis
18. Macrocyte
19, 20, 21. Variation in size and shape of the red blood cells
22. Polychromatophilia
23. Normoblast
24. Erythroblast

F. Infectious Mononucleosis

1. Bone marrow: normal
2. Red blood cell: normal
3. Volume of packed red blood cells: normal
4. Volume of packed white blood cells: normal
5. Plasma volume: normal
6. Normal red blood cell
7. Monocyte
8. Atypical lymphocyte
9. Lymphocyte
10. Neutrophil
11. Platelet

G. Chronic Lymphocytic Leukemia

1. Bone marrow: marrow infiltration, decrease in normal hematopoietic stem cells
2. Red blood cell: normal, increased regeneration
3. Volume of packed red blood cells: decreased
4. Volume of packed white blood cell: markedly increased
5. Plasma volume: slightly increased
6. Normal red bood cell
7, 8, 9. Variation in size and shape of the red blood cells
10. Polychromatophilia
11. Normoblast
12. Lymphoblast
13. Lymphocyte
14. Platelet

H. Chronic Myelocytic Leukemia

1. Bone marrow: marrow infiltration hyperplasia
2. Red blood cell: normal, increased regeneration
3. Volume of packed red blood cells: decreased
4. Volume of packed white blood cells: markedly increased
5. Plasma volume: increased
6. Normal red blood cell
7, 8, 9. Variation in size and shape of the red blood cells
10. Polychromatophilia
11. Myeloblast
12, 13. Neutrophilic myelocytes
14. Basophilic myelocyte
15. Eosinophilic myelocyte
16. Neutrophilic metamyelocyte
17. Eosinophilic metamyelocyte
18. Neutrophil
19. Eosinophil
20. Basophil
21. Platelet

I. Acute Leukemia

1. Bone marrow: marrow infiltration
2. Red blood cell: normal, increased regeneration
3. Volume of packed red blood cells: decreased
4. Volume of packed white blood cells: increased
5. Plasma volume: increased
6. Normal red blood cell
7, 8, 9. Variation in size and shape of red blood cells
10. Polychromatophilia
11. Normoblast
12. Stem cell
13. Lymphocyte
14. Platelet

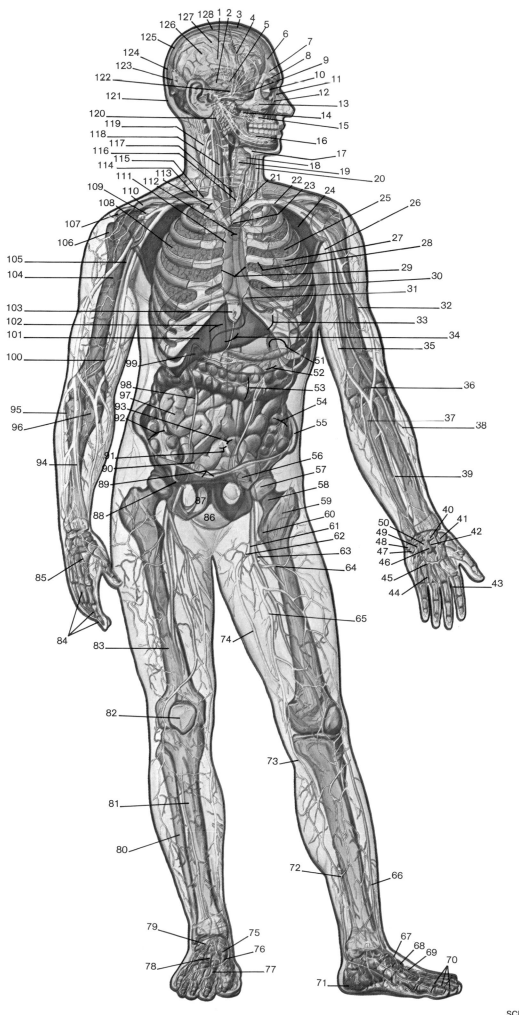

SCHICK-COLORPRINT® ANATOMY CHART
HUMAN BODY-FRONT
No. NS19 © 1988 AMERICAN MAP CORP.

HUMAN BODY - Front

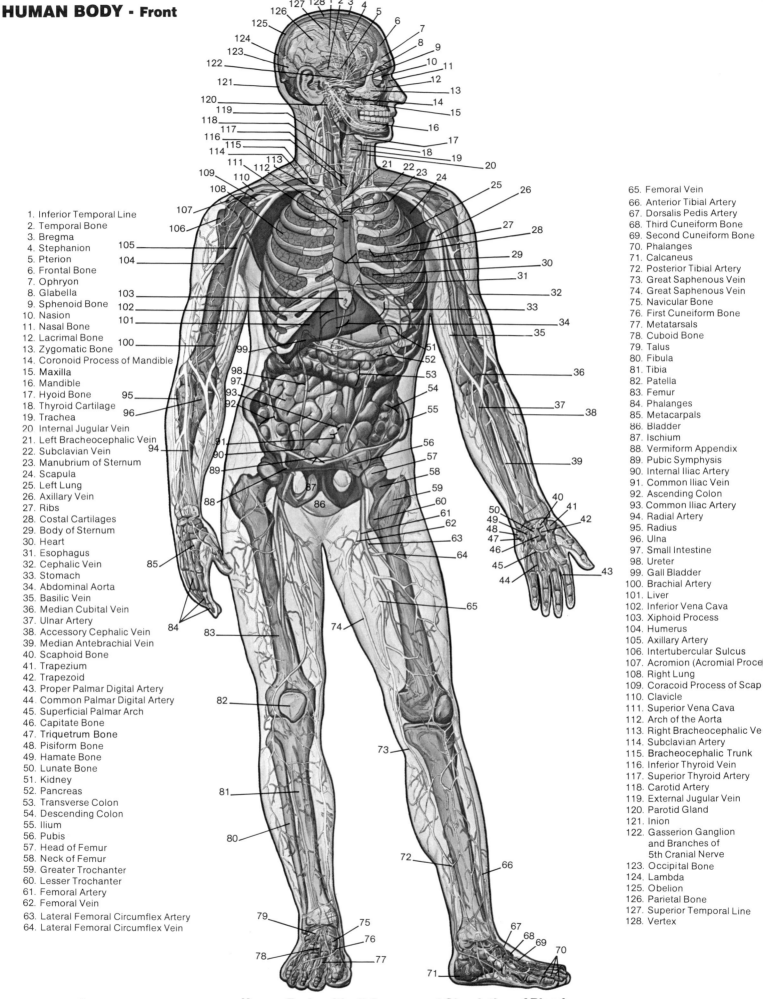

1. Inferior Temporal Line
2. Temporal Bone
3. Bregma
4. Stephanion
5. Pterion
6. Frontal Bone
7. Ophryon
8. Glabella
9. Sphenoid Bone
10. Nasion
11. Nasal Bone
12. Lacrimal Bone
13. Zygomatic Bone
14. Coronoid Process of Mandible
15. Maxilla
16. Mandible
17. Hyoid Bone
18. Thyroid Cartilage
19. Trachea
20. Internal Jugular Vein
21. Left Bracheocephalic Vein
22. Subclavian Vein
23. Manubrium of Sternum
24. Scapula
25. Left Lung
26. Axillary Vein
27. Ribs
28. Costal Cartilages
29. Body of Sternum
30. Heart
31. Esophagus
32. Cephalic Vein
33. Stomach
34. Abdominal Aorta
35. Basilic Vein
36. Median Cubital Vein
37. Ulnar Artery
38. Accessory Cephalic Vein
39. Median Antebrachial Vein
40. Scaphoid Bone
41. Trapezium
42. Trapezoid
43. Proper Palmar Digital Artery
44. Common Palmar Digital Artery
45. Superficial Palmar Arch
46. Capitate Bone
47. Triquetrum Bone
48. Pisiform Bone
49. Hamate Bone
50. Lunate Bone
51. Kidney
52. Pancreas
53. Transverse Colon
54. Descending Colon
55. Ilium
56. Pubis
57. Head of Femur
58. Neck of Femur
59. Greater Trochanter
60. Lesser Trochanter
61. Femoral Artery
62. Femoral Vein
63. Lateral Femoral Circumflex Artery
64. Lateral Femoral Circumflex Vein

65. Femoral Vein
66. Anterior Tibial Artery
67. Dorsalis Pedis Artery
68. Third Cuneiform Bone
69. Second Cuneiform Bone
70. Phalanges
71. Calcaneus
72. Posterior Tibial Artery
73. Great Saphenous Vein
74. Great Saphenous Vein
75. Navicular Bone
76. First Cuneiform Bone
77. Metatarsals
78. Cuboid Bone
79. Talus
80. Fibula
81. Tibia
82. Patella
83. Femur
84. Phalanges
85. Metacarpals
86. Bladder
87. Ischium
88. Vermiform Appendix
89. Pubic Symphysis
90. Internal Iliac Artery
91. Common Iliac Vein
92. Ascending Colon
93. Common Iliac Artery
94. Radial Artery
95. Radius
96. Ulna
97. Small Intestine
98. Ureter
99. Gall Bladder
100. Brachial Artery
101. Liver
102. Inferior Vena Cava
103. Xiphoid Process
104. Humerus
105. Axillary Artery
106. Intertubercular Sulcus
107. Acromion (Acromial Proce
108. Right Lung
109. Coracoid Process of Scap
110. Clavicle
111. Superior Vena Cava
112. Arch of the Aorta
113. Right Bracheocephalic Ve
114. Subclavian Artery
115. Bracheocephalic Trunk
116. Inferior Thyroid Vein
117. Superior Thyroid Artery
118. Carotid Artery
119. External Jugular Vein
120. Parotid Gland
121. Inion
122. Gasserion Ganglion
    and Branches of
    5th Cranial Nerve
123. Occipital Bone
124. Lambda
125. Obelion
126. Parietal Bone
127. Superior Temporal Line
128. Vertex

Human Body with all Organs and Circulation of Blood

SCHICK-COLORPRINT® ANATOMY CHART
HUMAN BODY-FRONT
No. NS19 © 1988 AMERICAN MAP CORP.

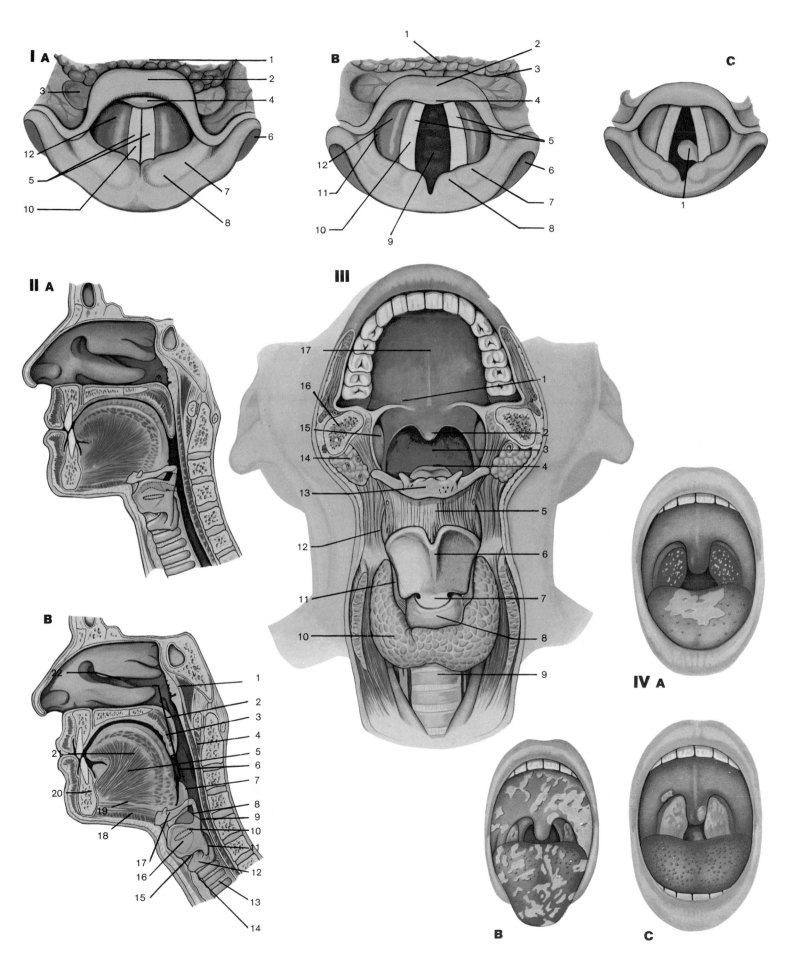

SCHICK-COLORPRINT®ANATOMY CHART
THE THROAT
No. NS20 © 1988 AMERICAN MAP CORP.

LARYNX WITH PHARYNX

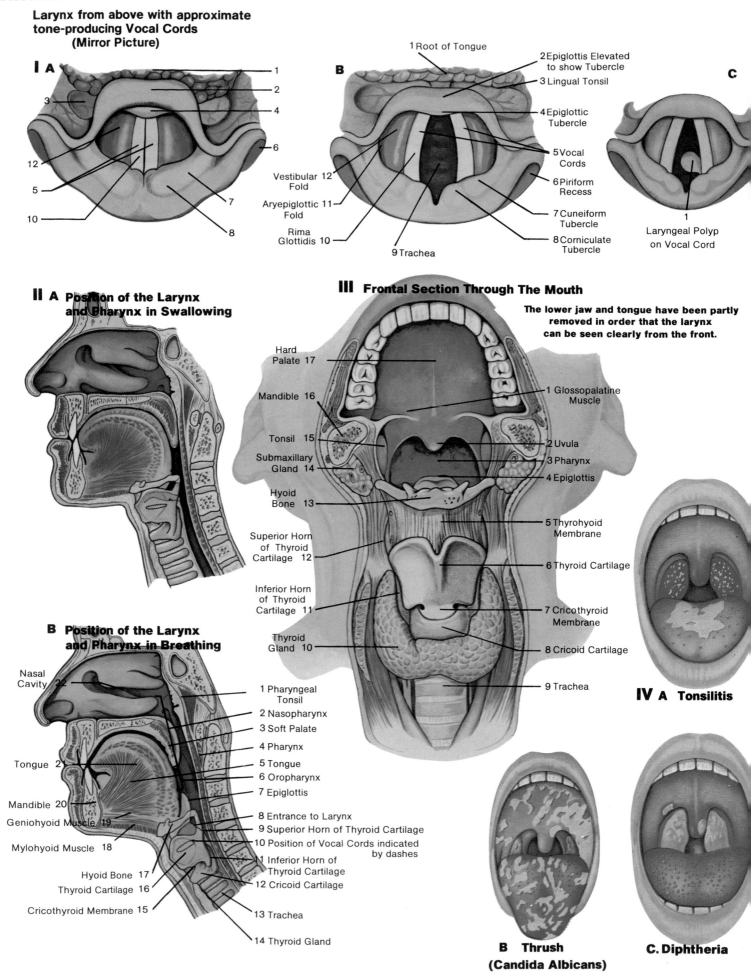

Larynx from above with approximate tone-producing Vocal Cords (Mirror Picture)

I A
1
2
3
4
12
6
5
10
7
8

B
1 Root of Tongue
2 Epiglottis Elevated to show Tubercle
3 Lingual Tonsil
4 Epiglottic Tubercle
5 Vocal Cords
6 Piriform Recess
7 Cuneiform Tubercle
8 Corniculate Tubercle
9 Trachea
Vestibular 12 Fold
Aryepiglottic 11 Fold
Rima Glottidis 10

C
1
Laryngeal Polyp on Vocal Cord

II A Position of the Larynx and Pharynx in Swallowing

III Frontal Section Through The Mouth

The lower jaw and tongue have been partly removed in order that the larynx can be seen clearly from the front.

Hard Palate 17
Mandible 16
Tonsil 15
Submaxillary Gland 14
Hyoid Bone 13
Superior Horn of Thyroid Cartilage 12
Inferior Horn of Thyroid Cartilage 11
Thyroid Gland 10

1 Glossopalatine Muscle
2 Uvula
3 Pharynx
4 Epiglottis
5 Thyrohyoid Membrane
6 Thyroid Cartilage
7 Cricothyroid Membrane
8 Cricoid Cartilage
9 Trachea

B Position of the Larynx and Pharynx in Breathing

Nasal Cavity 22
Tongue 21
Mandible 20
Geniohyoid Muscle 19
Mylohyoid Muscle 18
Hyoid Bone 17
Thyroid Cartilage 16
Cricothyroid Membrane 15

1 Pharyngeal Tonsil
2 Nasopharynx
3 Soft Palate
4 Pharynx
5 Tongue
6 Oropharynx
7 Epiglottis
8 Entrance to Larynx
9 Superior Horn of Thyroid Cartilage
10 Position of Vocal Cords indicated by dashes
11 Inferior Horn of Thyroid Cartilage
12 Cricoid Cartilage
13 Trachea
14 Thyroid Gland

IV A Tonsilitis

B Thrush (Candida Albicans)

C. Diphtheria

SCHICK-COLORPRINT® ANATOMY CHART
THE THROAT
No. NS20 © 1988 AMERICAN MAP CORP.

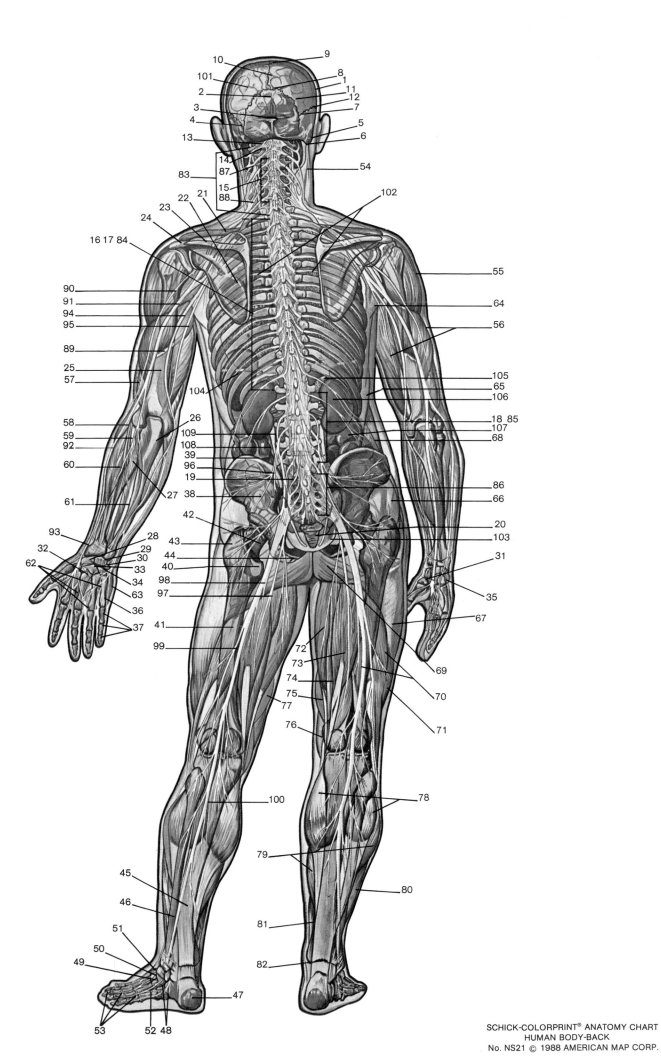

SCHICK-COLORPRINT® ANATOMY CHART
HUMAN BODY-BACK
No. NS21 © 1988 AMERICAN MAP CORP.

HUMAN BODY - Back

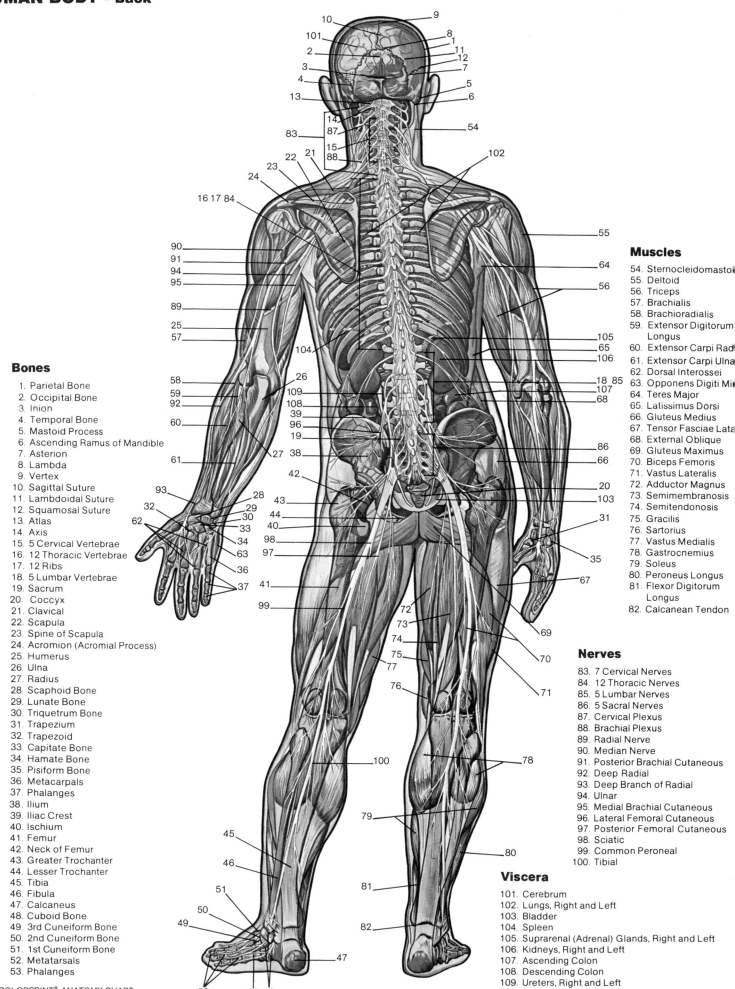

Bones

1. Parietal Bone
2. Occipital Bone
3. Inion
4. Temporal Bone
5. Mastoid Process
6. Ascending Ramus of Mandible
7. Asterion
8. Lambda
9. Vertex
10. Sagittal Suture
11. Lambdoidal Suture
12. Squamosal Suture
13. Atlas
14. Axis
15. 5 Cervical Vertebrae
16. 12 Thoracic Vertebrae
17. 12 Ribs
18. 5 Lumbar Vertebrae
19. Sacrum
20. Coccyx
21. Clavical
22. Scapula
23. Spine of Scapula
24. Acromion (Acromial Process)
25. Humerus
26. Ulna
27. Radius
28. Scaphoid Bone
29. Lunate Bone
30. Triquetrum Bone
31. Trapezium
32. Trapezoid
33. Capitate Bone
34. Hamate Bone
35. Pisiform Bone
36. Metacarpals
37. Phalanges
38. Ilium
39. Iliac Crest
40. Ischium
41. Femur
42. Neck of Femur
43. Greater Trochanter
44. Lesser Trochanter
45. Tibia
46. Fibula
47. Calcaneus
48. Cuboid Bone
49. 3rd Cuneiform Bone
50. 2nd Cuneiform Bone
51. 1st Cuneiform Bone
52. Metatarsals
53. Phalanges

Muscles

54. Sternocleidomasto[i]
55. Deltoid
56. Triceps
57. Brachialis
58. Brachioradialis
59. Extensor Digitorum Longus
60. Extensor Carpi Rad[ ]
61. Extensor Carpi Ulna[ ]
62. Dorsal Interossei
63. Opponens Digiti Mi[ ]
64. Teres Major
65. Latissimus Dorsi
66. Gluteus Medius
67. Tensor Fasciae Lata[ ]
68. External Oblique
69. Gluteus Maximus
70. Biceps Femoris
71. Vastus Lateralis
72. Adductor Magnus
73. Semimembranosis
74. Semitendonosis
75. Gracilis
76. Sartorius
77. Vastus Medialis
78. Gastrocnemius
79. Soleus
80. Peroneus Longus
81. Flexor Digitorum Longus
82. Calcanean Tendon

Nerves

83. 7 Cervical Nerves
84. 12 Thoracic Nerves
85. 5 Lumbar Nerves
86. 5 Sacral Nerves
87. Cervical Plexus
88. Brachial Plexus
89. Radial Nerve
90. Median Nerve
91. Posterior Brachial Cutaneous
92. Deep Radial
93. Deep Branch of Radial
94. Ulnar
95. Medial Brachial Cutaneous
96. Lateral Femoral Cutaneous
97. Posterior Femoral Cutaneous
98. Sciatic
99. Common Peroneal
100. Tibial

Viscera

101. Cerebrum
102. Lungs, Right and Left
103. Bladder
104. Spleen
105. Suprarenal (Adrenal) Glands, Right and Left
106. Kidneys, Right and Left
107. Ascending Colon
108. Descending Colon
109. Ureters, Right and Left

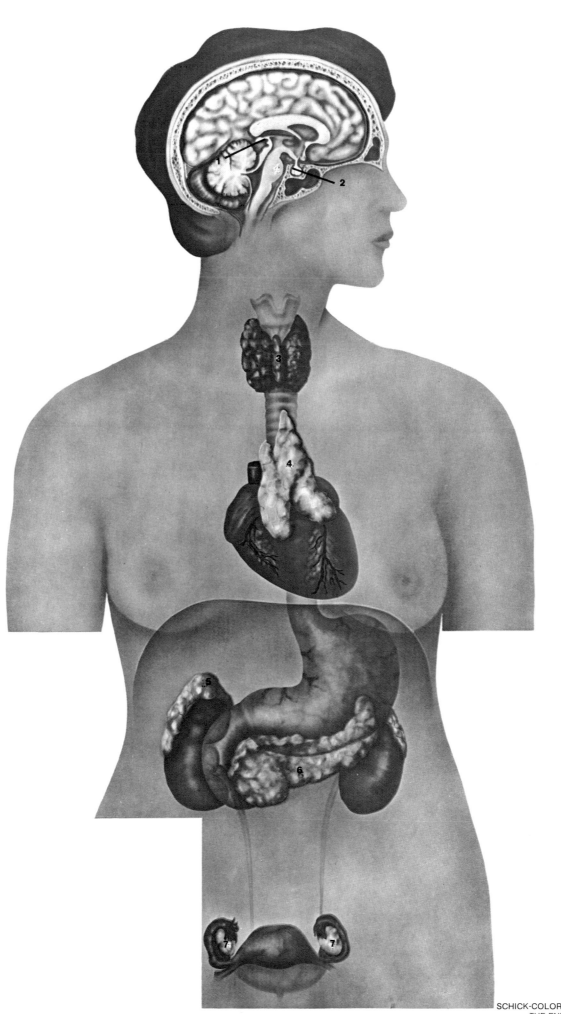

SCHICK-COLORPRINT® ANATOMY CHART
THE ENDOCRINE GLANDS
No. NS22 © 1988 AMERICAN MAP CORP.

ENDOCRINE GLANDS

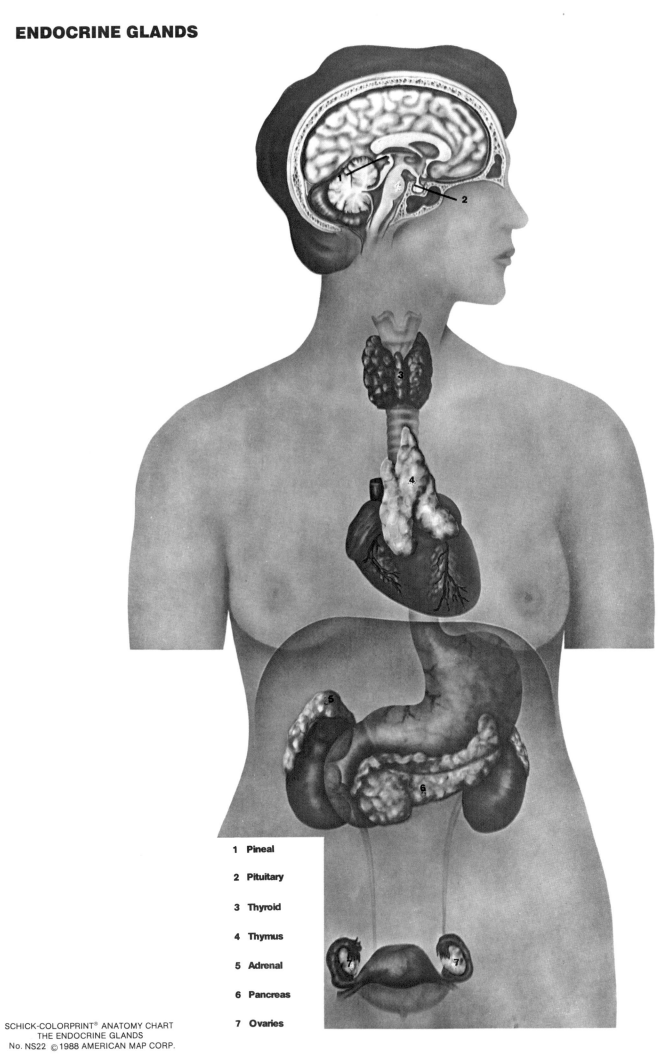

1 **Pineal**

2 **Pituitary**

3 **Thyroid**

4 **Thymus**

5 **Adrenal**

6 **Pancreas**

7 **Ovaries**

SCHICK-COLORPRINT® ANATOMY CHART
THE ENDOCRINE GLANDS
No. NS22 ©1988 AMERICAN MAP CORP.

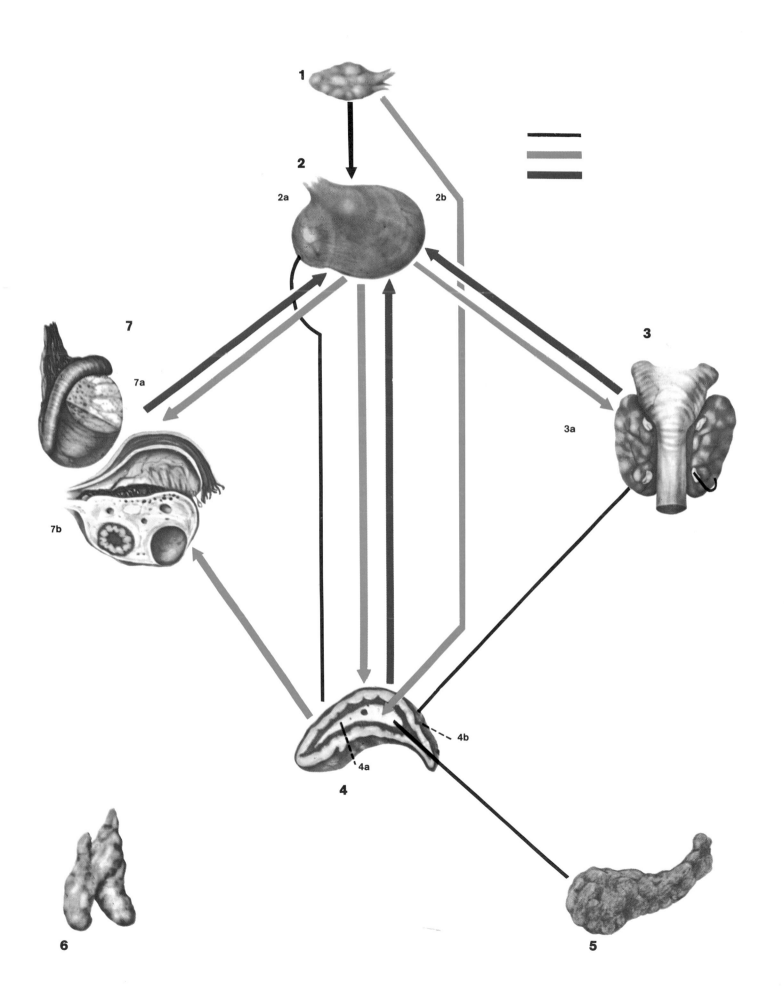

SCHICK-COLORPRINT® ANATOMY CHART
ENDOCRINE SYSTEM-INTERRELATIONS
No. NS23 ©1988 AMERICAN MAP CORP.

ENDOCRINE GLANDS
Diagram of Endocrine Interrelations

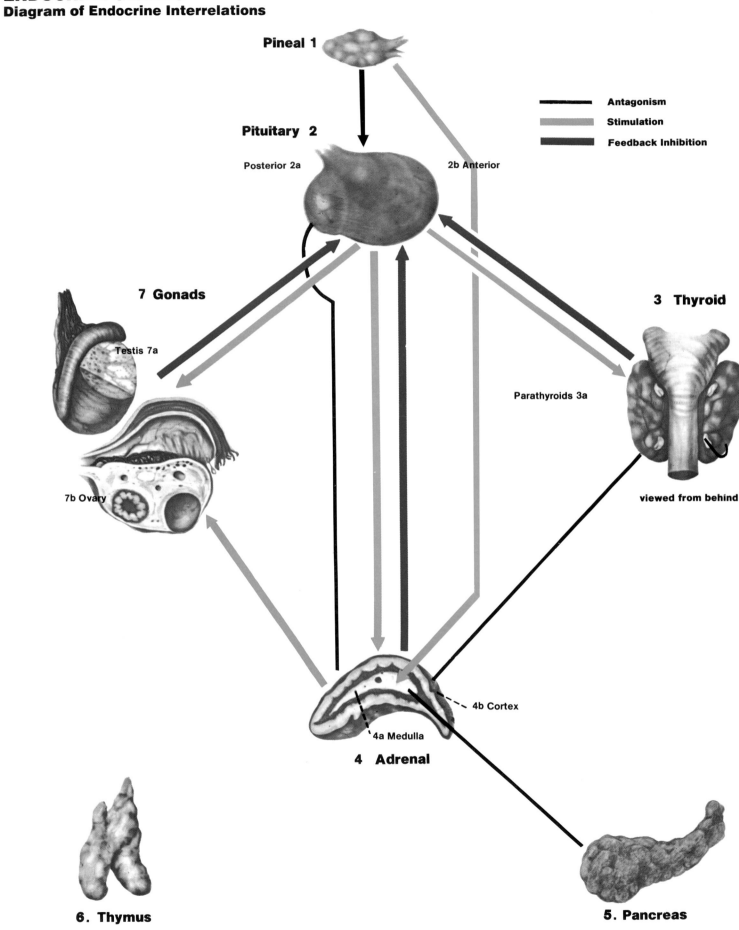

Pineal 1

Pituitary 2

Posterior 2a

2b Anterior

Antagonism
Stimulation
Feedback Inhibition

7 Gonads

Testis 7a

7b Ovary

3 Thyroid

Parathyroids 3a

viewed from behind

4b Cortex

4a Medulla

4 Adrenal

6. Thymus

5. Pancreas

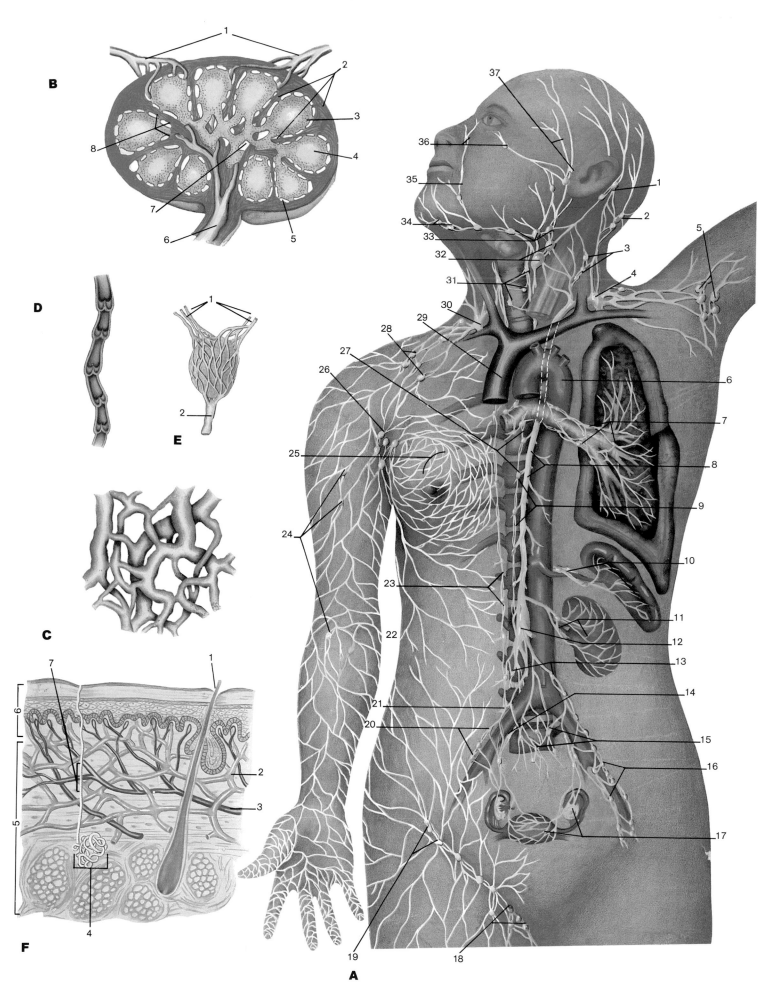

SCHICK-COLORPRINT® ANATOMY CHART
LYMPHATIC SYSTEM-GENERAL
NO. NS24 © 1988 AMERICAN MAP CORP.

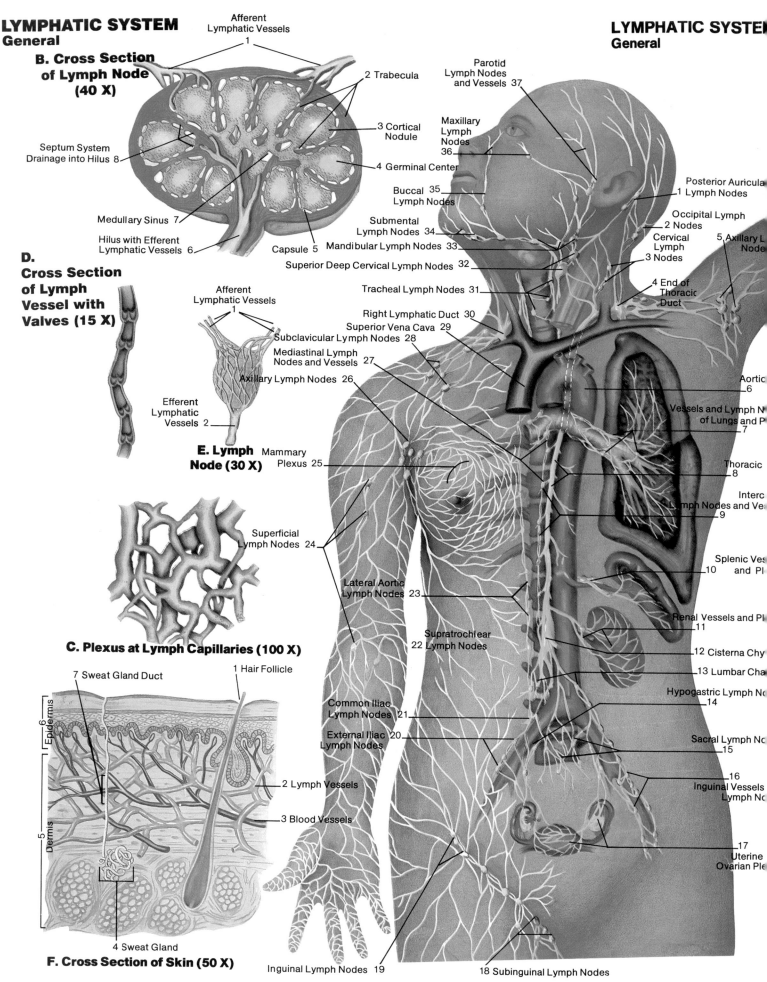

LYMPHATIC SYSTEM
General

B. Cross Section of Lymph Node (40 X)

Afferent Lymphatic Vessels 1

2 Trabecula

3 Cortical Nodule

4 Germinal Center

Septum System Drainage into Hilus 8

Medullary Sinus 7

Hilus with Efferent Lymphatic Vessels 6

Capsule 5

LYMPHATIC SYSTE
General

Parotid Lymph Nodes and Vessels 37

Maxillary Lymph Nodes 36

Buccal 35 Lymph Nodes

Submental Lymph Nodes 34

Mandibular Lymph Nodes 33

Superior Deep Cervical Lymph Nodes 32

Tracheal Lymph Nodes 31

Right Lymphatic Duct 30

Superior Vena Cava 29

Subclavicular Lymph Nodes 28

Mediastinal Lymph Nodes and Vessels 27

Axillary Lymph Nodes 26

Posterior Auricula 1 Lymph Nodes

Occipital Lymph 2 Nodes

Cervical Lymph 3 Nodes

4 End of Thoracic Duct

5 Axillary L Node

Aortic 6

Vessels and Lymph N of Lungs and P 7

Thoracic 8

Interc mph Nodes and Ve 9

Splenic Ves 10 and Pl

Renal Vessels and Pl 11

12 Cisterna Chy

13 Lumbar Cha

Hypogastric Lymph No 14

Sacral Lymph No 15

16 Inguinal Vessels Lymph No

17 Uterine Ovarian Ple

D. Cross Section of Lymph Vessel with Valves (15 X)

Afferent Lymphatic Vessels 1

Efferent Lymphatic Vessels 2

E. Lymph Node (30 X)

Mammary Plexus 25

Superficial Lymph Nodes 24

C. Plexus at Lymph Capillaries (100 X)

Lateral Aortic Lymph Nodes 23

Supratrochlear 22 Lymph Nodes

Common Iliac Lymph Nodes 21

External Iliac Lymph Nodes 20

7 Sweat Gland Duct

1 Hair Follicle

6 Epidermis

5 Dermis

2 Lymph Vessels

3 Blood Vessels

4 Sweat Gland

F. Cross Section of Skin (50 X)

Inguinal Lymph Nodes 19

18 Subinguinal Lymph Nodes

**A. All Superficial Lymph Nodes and Vessels in White.
All Deep Lymph Nodes and Vessels in Yellow.**

SCHICK-COLORPRINT® ANATOMY CHART
LYMPHATIC SYSTEM-GENERAL
NO. NS24 © 1988 AMERICAN MAP CORP.

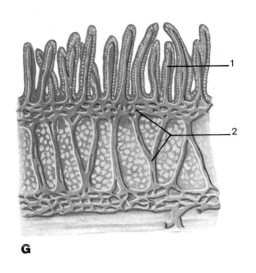

G

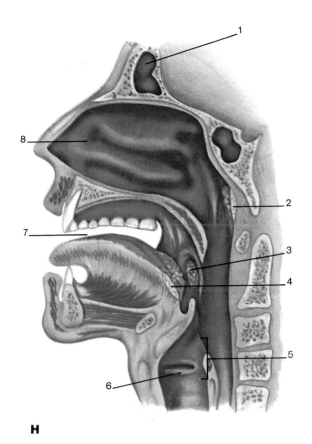

H

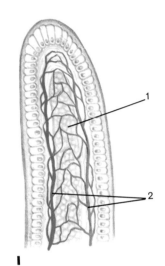

I

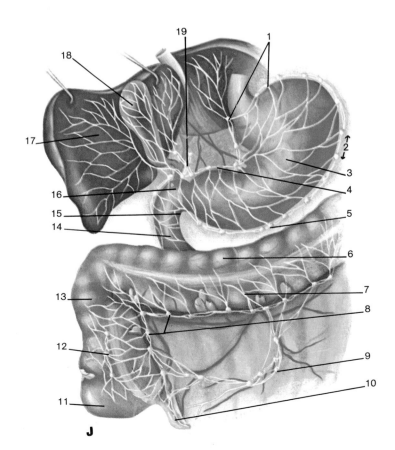

J

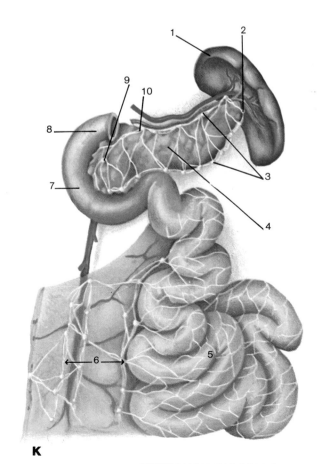

K

LYMPHATIC SYSTEM
Nodes and Vessels

All Superficial Lymph Nodes and Vessels in White
All Deep Lymph Nodes and Vessels in Yellow

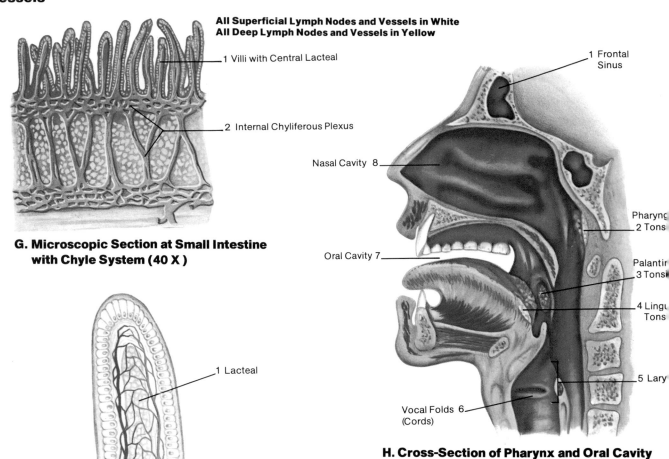

1 Villi with Central Lacteal

2 Internal Chyliferous Plexus

G. Microscopic Section at Small Intestine with Chyle System (40 X)

1 Lacteal

2 Artery and Vein

I. Intestinal Villus

1 Frontal Sinus

Nasal Cavity 8

Oral Cavity 7

Pharyng 2 Tons

Palantir 3 Tons

4 Lingu Tons

5 Lary

Vocal Folds 6 (Cords)

H. Cross-Section of Pharynx and Oral Cavity

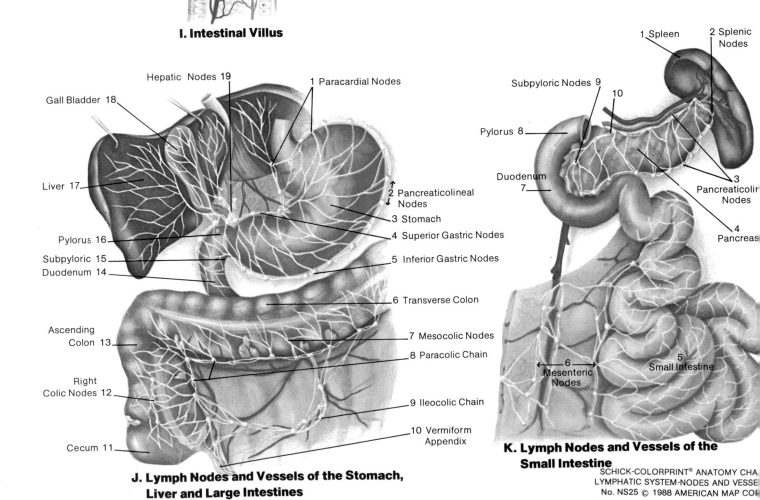

Hepatic Nodes 19

Gall Bladder 18

1 Paracardial Nodes

Liver 17

2 Pancreaticolineal Nodes

3 Stomach

4 Superior Gastric Nodes

Pylorus 16

Subpyloric 15

Duodenum 14

5 Inferior Gastric Nodes

6 Transverse Colon

Ascending Colon 13

7 Mesocolic Nodes

8 Paracolic Chain

Right Colic Nodes 12

9 Ileocolic Chain

10 Vermiform Appendix

Cecum 11

J. Lymph Nodes and Vessels of the Stomach, Liver and Large Intestines

1 Spleen

2 Splenic Nodes

Subpyloric Nodes 9

10

Pylorus 8

Duodenum 7

3 Pancreaticolin Nodes

4 Pancreas

6 Mesenteric Nodes

5 Small Intestine

K. Lymph Nodes and Vessels of the Small Intestine

SCHICK-COLORPRINT® ANATOMY CHA
LYMPHATIC SYSTEM-NODES AND VESSE
No. NS25 © 1988 AMERICAN MAP CO

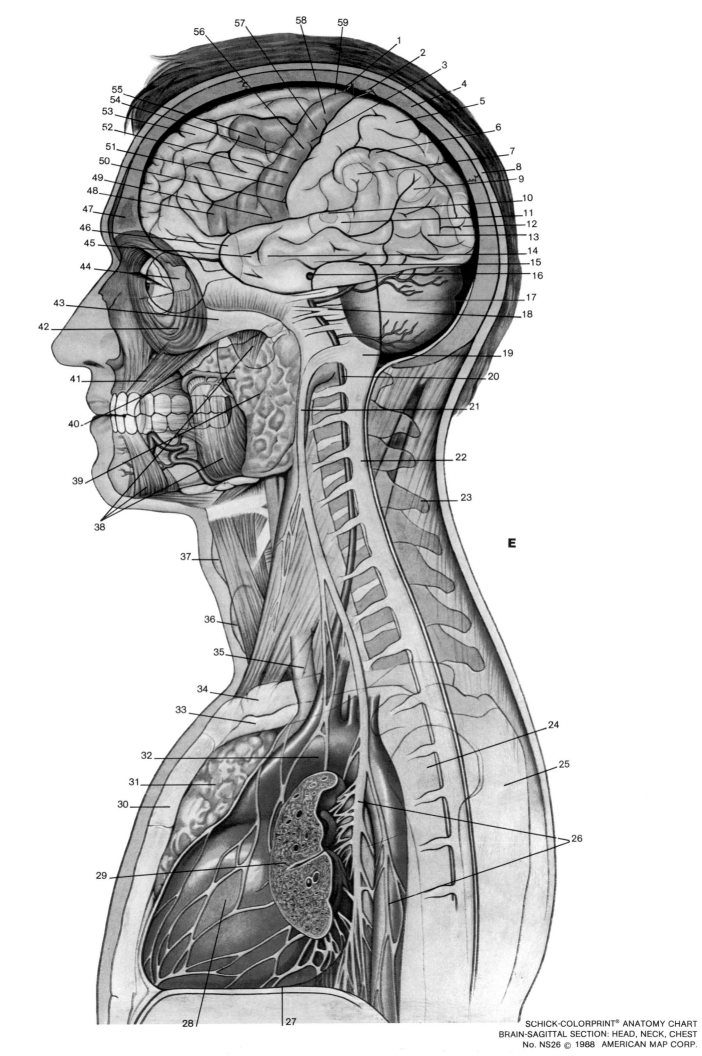

56 57   58   59
                              1
55   2
54   3
53   4
52   5
                                6
51   7
50   8
49   9
48   10
47   11
46   12
45   13
                                14
44   15
                                16
43
42   17
                                18

41   19

40   20

                                21
39
                                22

                                23
38
                                        E

37

36   24

35   25

34
33

32

31
                                        26
30

29

                              28   27

SCHICK-COLORPRINT® ANATOMY CHART
BRAIN-SAGITTAL SECTION: HEAD, NECK, CHEST
No. NS26 © 1988 AMERICAN MAP CORP.

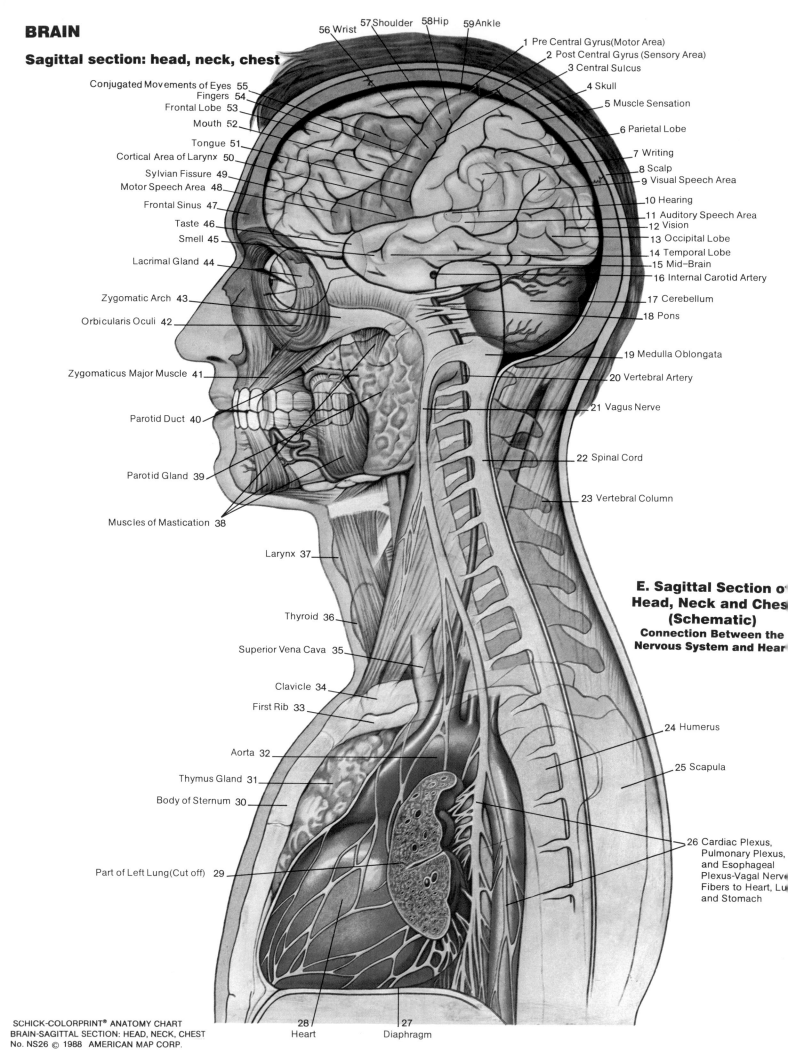

BRAIN

Sagittal section: head, neck, chest

56 Wrist 57 Shoulder 58 Hip 59 Ankle

1 Pre Central Gyrus(Motor Area)
2 Post Central Gyrus (Sensory Area)
3 Central Sulcus
4 Skull
5 Muscle Sensation
6 Parietal Lobe
7 Writing
8 Scalp
9 Visual Speech Area
10 Hearing
11 Auditory Speech Area
12 Vision
13 Occipital Lobe
14 Temporal Lobe
15 Mid-Brain
16 Internal Carotid Artery
17 Cerebellum
18 Pons
19 Medulla Oblongata
20 Vertebral Artery
21 Vagus Nerve
22 Spinal Cord
23 Vertebral Column

24 Humerus
25 Scapula
26 Cardiac Plexus, Pulmonary Plexus, and Esophageal Plexus-Vagal Nerve Fibers to Heart, Lung and Stomach

Conjugated Movements of Eyes 55
Fingers 54
Frontal Lobe 53
Mouth 52
Tongue 51
Cortical Area of Larynx 50
Sylvian Fissure 49
Motor Speech Area 48
Frontal Sinus 47
Taste 46
Smell 45
Lacrimal Gland 44
Zygomatic Arch 43
Orbicularis Oculi 42
Zygomaticus Major Muscle 41
Parotid Duct 40
Parotid Gland 39
Muscles of Mastication 38
Larynx 37
Thyroid 36
Superior Vena Cava 35
Clavicle 34
First Rib 33
Aorta 32
Thymus Gland 31
Body of Sternum 30
Part of Left Lung(Cut off) 29

28 Heart
27 Diaphragm

E. Sagittal Section of Head, Neck and Chest (Schematic)
Connection Between the Nervous System and Heart

SCHICK-COLORPRINT® ANATOMY CHART
BRAIN-SAGITTAL SECTION: HEAD, NECK, CHEST
No. NS26 © 1988 AMERICAN MAP CORP.

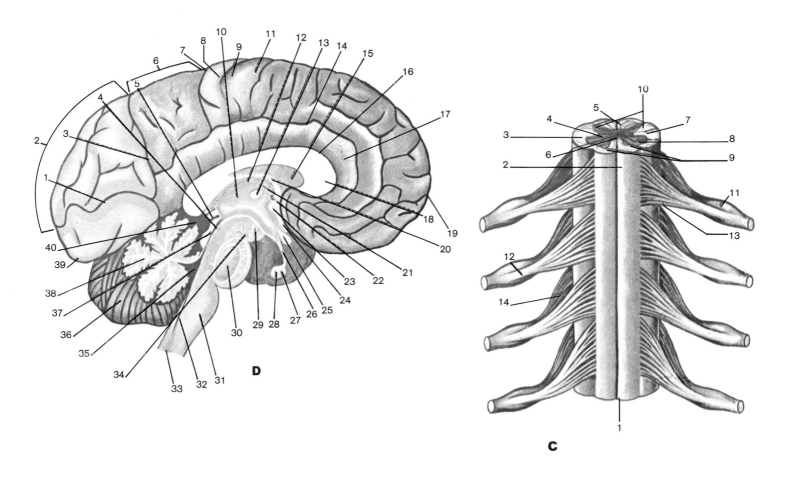

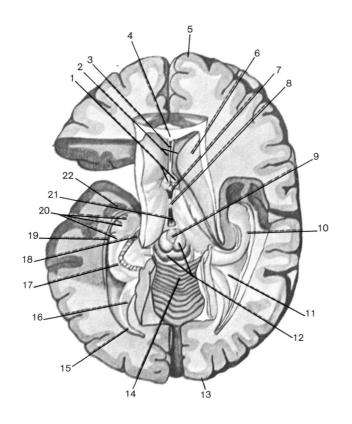

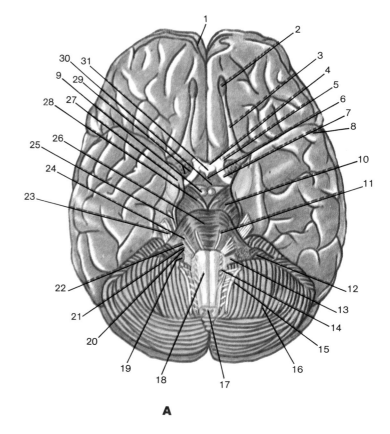

SCHICK-COLORPRINT® ANATOMY CHART
BRAIN-MEDIAN SAGITTAL AND HORIZONTAL SECTIONS, SPINAL CORD, BASE OF BRAIN
No. NS27 © 1988 AMERICAN MAP CORP.

Brain
Median sagittal and horizontal sections, spinal cord, base of brain

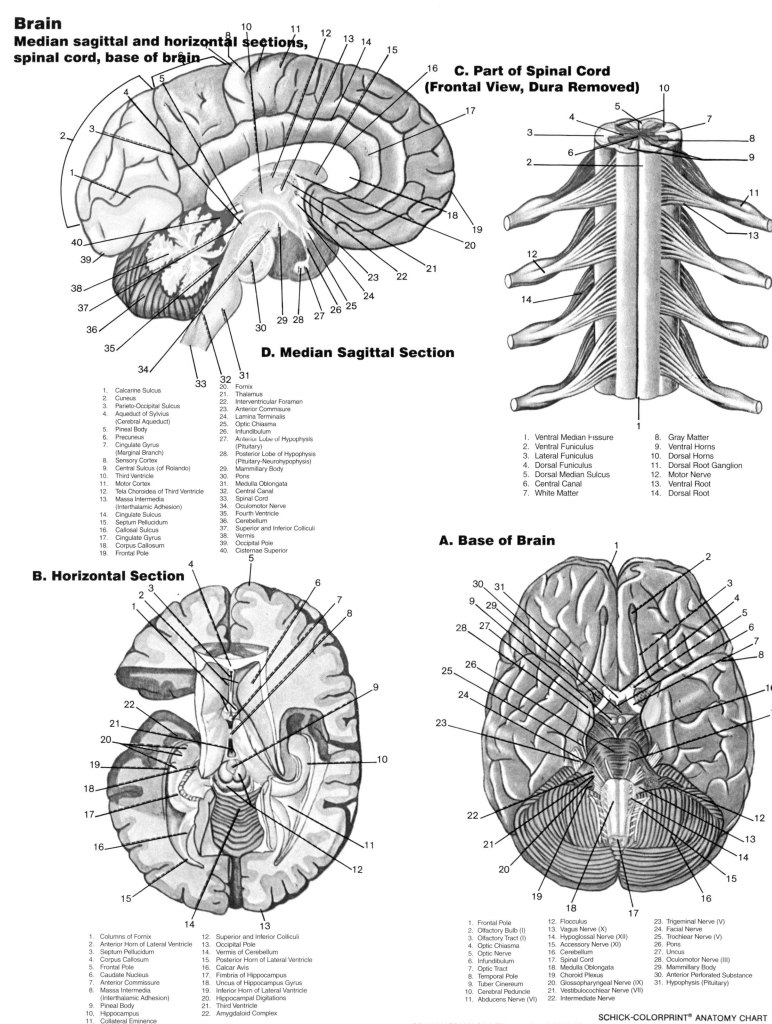

C. Part of Spinal Cord (Frontal View, Dura Removed)

D. Median Sagittal Section

1. Calcarine Sulcus
2. Cuneus
3. Parieto-Occipital Sulcus
4. Aqueduct of Sylvius (Cerebral Aqueduct)
5. Pineal Body
6. Precuneus
7. Cingulate Gyrus (Marginal Branch)
8. Sensory Cortex
9. Central Sulcus (of Rolando)
10. Third Ventricle
11. Motor Cortex
12. Tela Choroidea of Third Ventricle
13. Massa Intermedia (Interthalamic Adhesion)
14. Cingulate Sulcus
15. Septum Pellucidum
16. Callosal Sulcus
17. Cingulate Gyrus
18. Corpus Callosum
19. Frontal Pole
20. Fornix
21. Thalamus
22. Interventricular Foramen
23. Anterior Commisure
24. Lamina Terminalis
25. Optic Chiasma
26. Infundibulum
27. Anterior Lobe of Hypophysis (Pituitary)
28. Posterior Lobe of Hypophysis (Pituitary-Neurohypophysis)
29. Mammillary Body
30. Pons
31. Medulla Oblongata
32. Central Canal
33. Spinal Cord
34. Oculomotor Nerve
35. Fourth Ventricle
36. Cerebellum
37. Superior and Inferior Colliculi
38. Vermis
39. Occipital Pole
40. Cisternae Superior

Spinal cord legend:

1. Ventral Median Fissure
2. Ventral Funiculus
3. Lateral Funiculus
4. Dorsal Funiculus
5. Dorsal Median Sulcus
6. Central Canal
7. White Matter
8. Gray Matter
9. Ventral Horns
10. Dorsal Horns
11. Dorsal Root Ganglion
12. Motor Nerve
13. Ventral Root
14. Dorsal Root

B. Horizontal Section

1. Columns of Fornix
2. Anterior Horn of Lateral Ventricle
3. Septum Pellucidum
4. Corpus Callosum
5. Frontal Pole
6. Caudate Nucleus
7. Anterior Commissure
8. Massa Intermedia (Interthalamic Adhesion)
9. Pineal Body
10. Hippocampus
11. Collateral Eminence
12. Superior and Inferior Colliculi
13. Occipital Pole
14. Vermis of Cerebellum
15. Posterior Horn of Lateral Ventricle
16. Calcar Avis
17. Fimbria of Hippocampus
18. Uncus of Hippocampus Gyrus
19. Inferior Horn of Lateral Vantricle
20. Hippocampal Digitations
21. Third Ventricle
22. Amygdaloid Complex

A. Base of Brain

1. Frontal Pole
2. Olfactory Bulb (I)
3. Olfactory Tract (I)
4. Optic Chiasma
5. Optic Nerve
6. Infundibulum
7. Optic Tract
8. Temporal Pole
9. Tuber Cinereum
10. Cerebral Peduncle
11. Abducens Nerve (VI)
12. Flocculus
13. Vagus Nerve (X)
14. Hypoglossal Nerve (XII)
15. Accessory Nerve (XI)
16. Cerebellum
17. Spinal Cord
18. Medulla Oblongata
19. Choroid Plexus
20. Glossopharyngeal Nerve (IX)
21. Vestibulocochlear Nerve (VII)
22. Intermediate Nerve
23. Trigeminal Nerve (V)
24. Facial Nerve
25. Trochlear Nerve (V)
26. Pons
27. Uncus
28. Oculomotor Nerve (III)
29. Mammillary Body
30. Anterior Perforated Substance
31. Hypophysis (Pituitary)

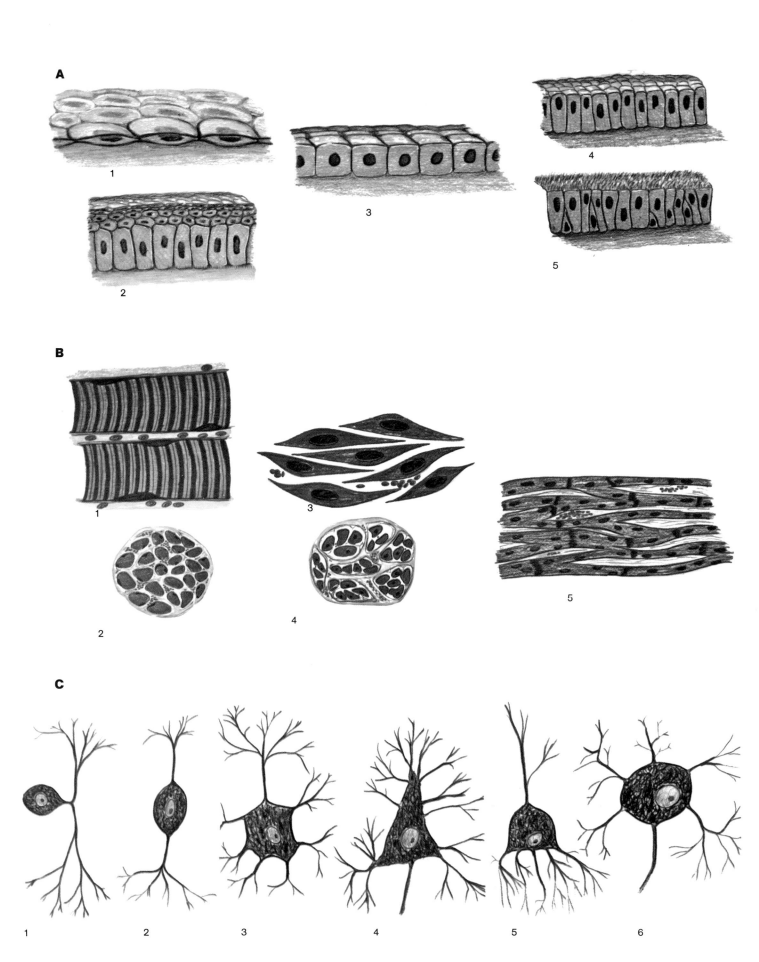

A

1

2

3

4

5

B

1

2

3

4

5

C

1

2

3

4

5

6

TISSUES

A Epithelial Tissue

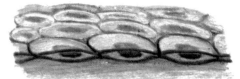

1 Simple Squamous

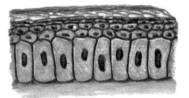

3 Cuboidal

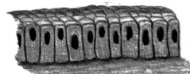

4 Simple Columnar

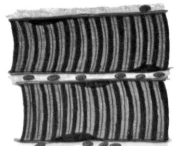

2 Stratified Squamous

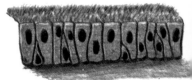

5 Pseudostratified Columnar Ciliated

B Muscular Tissue

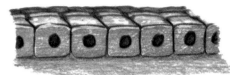

1 Skeletal Muscle Cells

Smooth Muscle Cells

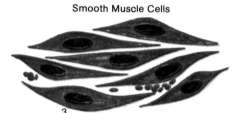

3

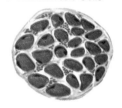

2 Bundles of Skeletal Muscles

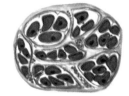

4 Bundles of Smooth Muscles

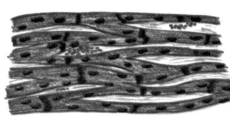

5 Cardiac Muscle Cells

C Nervous Tissue

Various Types of Neurons

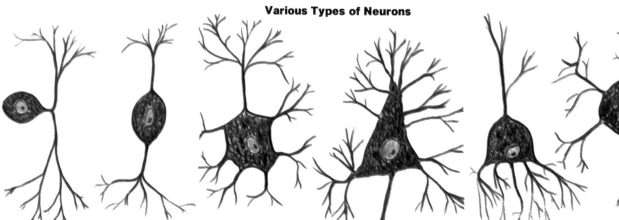

1 Pseudounipolar   2 Bipolar   3 Multipolar   4 Pyramidal Cell   5 Purkinje Cell   6 Autonomic Ganglion Cell

SCHICK-COLORPRINT® ANATOMY CHART
TISSUES
No. NS28 ©1988 AMERICAN MAP CORP

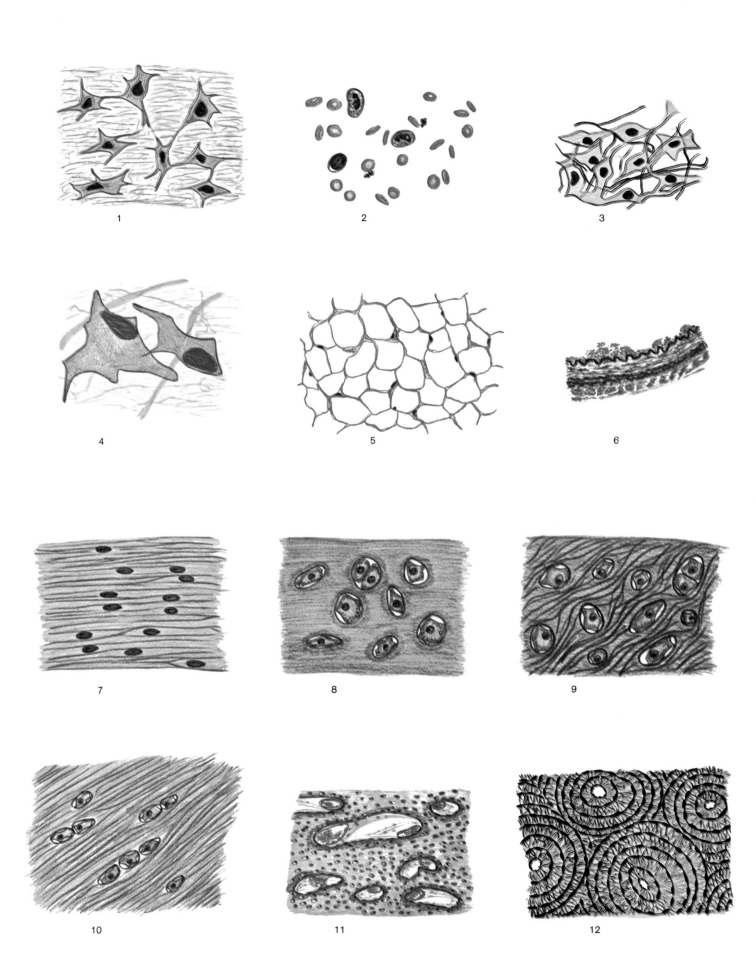

1

2

3

4

5

6

7

8

9

10

11

12

SCHICK-COLORPRINT® ANATOMY CHART
TISSUES
No.NS29 ©1988 AMERICAN MAP CORP.

TISSUES

Connective Tissue

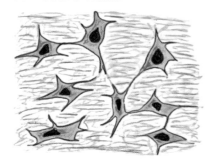

1 Mesenchymal

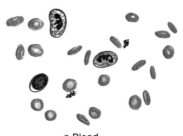

2 Blood

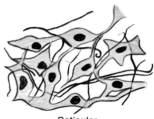

3 Reticular

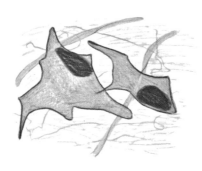

4 Areolar (Loose)

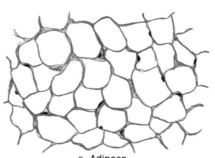

5 Adipose

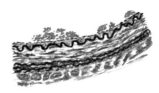

6 Elastic

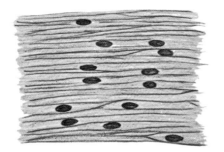

7 Fibrous (Dense)

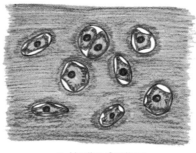

8 Hyaline Cartilage

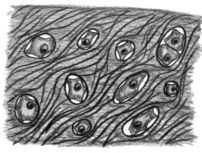

9 Elastic Cartilage

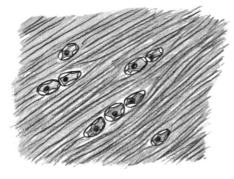

10 Fibrocartilage

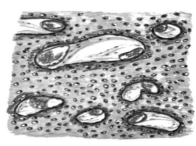

11 Cancellous Bone

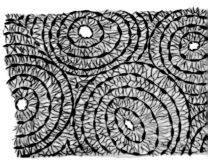

12 Compact Bone

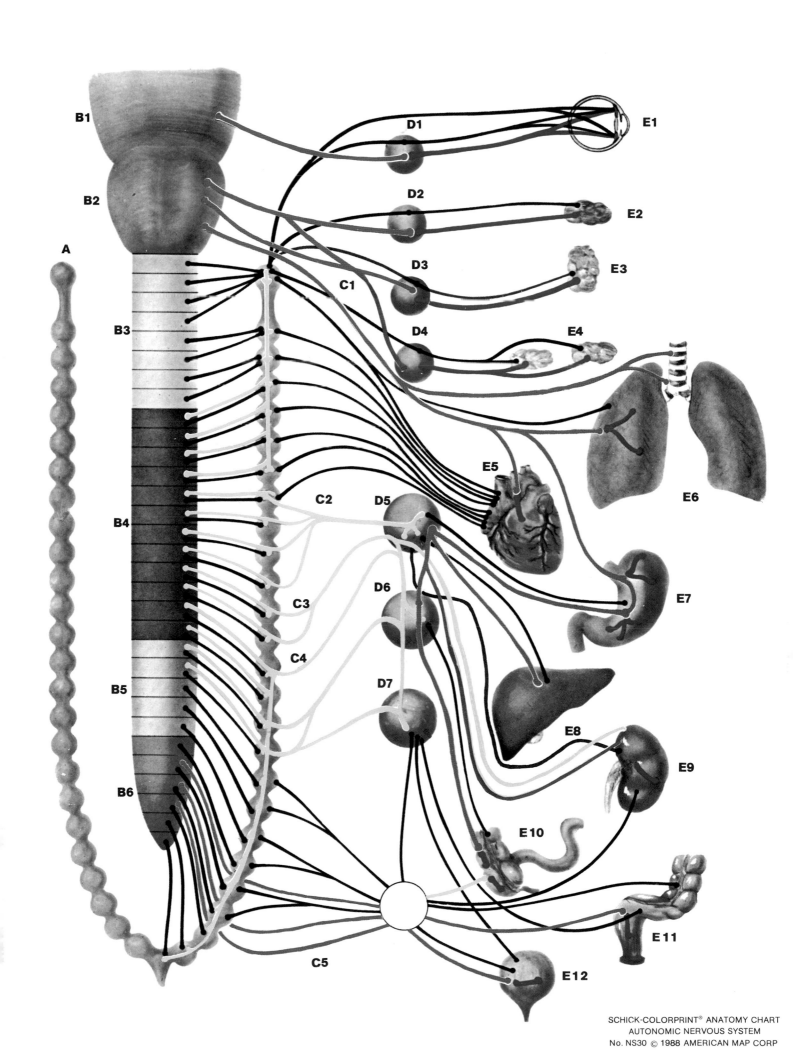

AUTONOMIC NERVOUS SYSTEM

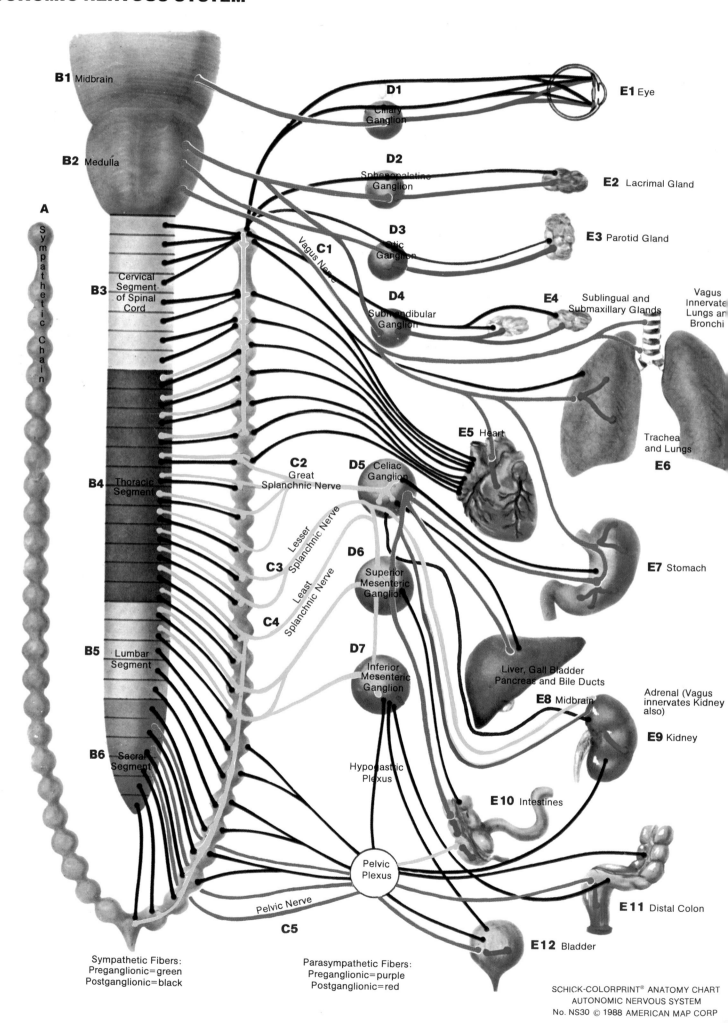

B1 Midbrain

B2 Medulla

A Sympathetic Chain

B3 Cervical Segment of Spinal Cord

B4 Thoracic Segment

B5 Lumbar Segment

B6 Sacral Segment

C1 Vagus Nerve

C2 Great Splanchnic Nerve

C3 Lesser Splanchnic Nerve

C4 Least Splanchnic Nerve

C5 Pelvic Nerve

Hypogastric Plexus

Pelvic Plexus

D1 Ciliary Ganglion

D2 Sphenopalatine Ganglion

D3 Otic Ganglion

D4 Submandibular Ganglion

D5 Celiac Ganglion

D6 Superior Mesenteric Ganglion

D7 Inferior Mesenteric Ganglion

E1 Eye

E2 Lacrimal Gland

E3 Parotid Gland

E4 Sublingual and Submaxillary Glands

Vagus Innervate Lungs and Bronchi

E5 Heart

Trachea and Lungs

E6

E7 Stomach

Liver, Gall Bladder Pancreas and Bile Ducts

E8 Midbrain

Adrenal (Vagus innervates Kidney also)

E9 Kidney

E10 Intestines

E11 Distal Colon

E12 Bladder

Sympathetic Fibers:
Preganglionic=green
Postganglionic=black

Parasympathetic Fibers:
Preganglionic=purple
Postganglionic=red

SCHICK-COLORPRINT® ANATOMY CHART
AUTONOMIC NERVOUS SYSTEM
No. NS30 © 1988 AMERICAN MAP CORP

Colorprint®-Schick Anatomy Atlas
Index

Anatomical Feature	Chart number, bold Feature number, light	Anatomical Feature	Chart number, bold Feature number, light
A		ARTERIES (Continued)	
Abdominal Wall	**10**-D8	Epigastric	
Acromion (Acromial Process)	**1**-12; **19**-107; **21**-24	Superficial	**1**-66
Adipose Tissue	**29**-5	Superior	**1**-58
Adrenal Glands	**10**-D3,D24; **21**-105; **22**-5; **23**-4	of Eye	**2**-A8
Afferent Vessels (Lymph Node)	**24**-B1,	Facial	**1**-49
ALVEOLUS (ALVEOLI)		Femoral	**1**-72 ;**19**-61
Capillary Network	**17**-A1,A9	Genicular, descending	**1**-73
Carbon Dioxide is Expired	**17**-A6	Gonadal	**10**-D21
Cross Section	**17**-A2	Iliac	
Oxygen passes through	**17**-A7	Common	**10**-D10 **19**-93
Amnion	**11**-H5	with Common Iliac Vein	**13**-A1; **19**-91
Amnion Cavity	**11**-H6	External	**1**-65;**10**-D12
AMPULLA		Internal	**1**-64;**10**-D11;**19**-90
of Ear	**9**-A26,B2,B9	Intercostal	**1**-59
of Vas	**13**-A24	Interlobular, of Kidney	**10**-C6
Amygdaloid Complex of Brain	**27**-B22	Interosseous	**1**-67
ANASTOMOSIS		of Intestinal Villus	**6**-C3
Circumpatellar	**1**-75	of Kidney (renal)	**10**-A13
Around Elbow Joint	**1**-61	Palmar Arches, Superficial	
ANEMIA		and Deep	**1**-69
Congenital Hemolytic	**18**-D	Perforating, of Kidney	**10**-C3
Erythroblastosis Fetalis	**18**-E18 to E24	Peroneal	**1**-78
Lead Poisoning	**18**-E6-E12	Plantar Arch	**1**-82
Megaloblastic Anemia		Popliteal	**1**-76
(Pernicious Anemia)	**18**-B	Pressure Points of	
Microcytic Hypochromic Anemia		Main Arteries	**1**
(Iron Deficiency)	**18**-C	Profunda (Femoris)	**1**-71
Sickle Cell	**18**-E13 to E17	Pulmonary	**1**-54; **4**-A30,B12; **7**-23
Antrum, Pyloric	**5**-24	Left Main Branch	**4**-D3
Anus	**12**-A15,C5	Radial	**19**-94
Apex of Heart	**4**-A21	Renal	**10**-A13
Apical Spiral of Ear	**9**-B5	Ramification of	**10**-A5
Appendix	**5**-34; **19**-88; **25**-J10	of Skin	**3**-16,26,29
Appendices Epiploicae	**5**-31	Subclavian	**1**-51; **19**-114
Aqueduct of Sylvius	**27**-D4	Left	**4**-A7
ARCH		Right	**4**-A2
Aortic	**1**-53;**4**-A8;**19**-112;**24**-A6	Temporal, Superficial	**1**-47
Superior Branches	**4**-D1	Thoracic, Internal	**1**-55
Bracheocephalic	**4**-D1a	Thyroid, Superior	**19**-117
Left Common Carotid	**4**-D1b	Tibial	
Left Subclavian	**4**-D1c	Anterior	**1**-79; **19**-66
Branchial	**11**-K2	Posterior	**1**-77; **19**-72
Hyoid	**20**-IIB17	Ulnar	**1**-63; **19**-37
Palmar, Superficial	**19**-45	Vertebral	**26**-20
Plantar	**1**-82	Asterion	**21**-7
Areolar Tissue	**29**-4	Atlas	**21**-13
ARTERIES		Atrium of Heart	
Arteries	**1**-47-84; **3**-16,26,29	Left	**4**-A12,D5,C4
Anastomosis Around Elbow	**1**-61	Right	**4**-A29,C6
Aorta	**4**-B1,D2; **7**-22; **26**-32	Auricle	
Abdominal	**1**-60; **10**-D9; **19**-34	Left	**4**-B11,D6
Arch of	**1**-53; **4**-A8; **19**-112; **24**-A6	Right	**4**-D10
Superior Branches	**4**-D1	Auricular Lymph Nodes	
Bracheocephalic	**4**-D1a	Posterior	**24**-A1
Left Common Carotid	**4**-D1b	AUTONOMIC NERVOUS SYSTEM	
Left Subclavion	**4**-D1c	Autonomic Nervous System	**30**
Descending	**4**-A20	Parasympathetic Fibers	**30**
Arcuate	**1**-81; **10**-C9	Sympathetic Chain	**30**-A
Axillary	**1**-52; **19**-105	Sympathetic Fibers	**30**
Bracheocephalic Trunk	**19**-115	Axillary Lymph Nodes	**16**-6; **24**-A5,A26
Brachial	**1**-57; **19**-100	Axis	**21**-14
Circumpatellar Anastomosis	**1**-75		
Carotid	**19**-118		
Common	**1**-50	**B**	
Left	**4**-A6	BACTERIA	
Right	**4**-A5	on Foreign Body	**17**-B2
External	**1**-48	White Cells Moving Toward	**17**-B3
Internal	**9**-A16;**26**-16	BASOPHIL	
Carpal, Dorsal Ulnar	**1**-68	Mature	**16**-23
Circumflex, Lateral		Normal Quantity	**17** NBC
Descending Branch of	**1**-74	Biceps Femoris	**21**-70
Circumflex, Lateral Femoral	**19**-63	BLADDER	
Digital		Gall	**5**-45;**19**-99;**25**-J18;**30**-E8
Common Palmar	**1**-84;**19**-44	Urinary	**10**-D13;**12**-A8; **13**-B3; **19**-86 ; **21**-103;**30**-E12
First Dorsal Interosseus	**1**-70	Apex	**13**-A6c
Proper Palmar	**19**-43	Body	**13**-A6a
Dorsalis Pedis	**1**-80; **19**-67		

Anatomical Feature	Chart number, bold Feature number, light	Anatomical Feature	Chart number, bold Feature number, light
BLADDER (Continued)		BLOOD CELLS (Continued)	
Neck	13-A6b	Variation	
BLOOD	16;17;18	Size and Shape	18-B7 to B9,C7 to C9, D8 to D10,E8 to E10, E19 to E21,G7 to G9, H7 to H9,I7 to I9
Circulation	19		
Diseases of Blood Cells	18		
Groups, Compatibility of	17-D		
Donor	17-D2	Volume	18-B,C,D,E,G,H,I(3)
Recipient	17-D1	Vessels	11-H2
Liquid Connective Tissue	29-2	Reticulocyte	16-18
Normal	18-A	Sickle Cell	18-E13
Normal Blood Cell Volume	17-E	Sickle Cell Anemia	18-E13 to E17
Erythrocytes	17-E3	White	
Leukocytes	17-E2	Function	17-B
Plasma	17-E1	Moving toward Bacteria	17-B3
Normal Blood Counts	17	Normal Count	17-NBC
Plasma	18-A,B,C,D,E,F,G,H,I(5)	Mature	
Venous, moving through Capillary	17-A4	Basophilic	16-23;18-H20
Vessels	4-D4;11-H2 13-B14,A19;24-F3	Eosinophilic	16-22;18-A8,H19
		Migration through Capillary Wall	17-C3
See also Blood Cells		Neutrophilic	16-21;18-A7,B11,C10,D11,E11 E16,F10,H18
BLOOD CELLS	16;17;18		
Development of	16	Unsegmented	18-D12
Diseases of		Volume	
Anemia		Normal	17-E;18-A,C,D,E,F(4)
Congenital Hemolytic	18-D	Variation in	18-B,C,D,E,F,G,H,I (3,4)
Megaloblastic	18-B	BODY, HUMAN	
Microcytic Hypochromic	18-C	Back View with Bones, Muscles,	
Special Forms	18-E	Nerves, Viscera	21
Erythroblastosis Fetalis	18-E18 to E24	Front View	
Lead Poisoning	18-E6-E12	Bones and Arteries	1
Sickle Cell	18-E13 to E17	Digestive System	5
Infectious Mononucleosis	18-F	Endocrine Glands	22
		Lymphatic System	24-A
Leukemia		Organs and Circulation	19
Acute	18-I	BONE MARROW	
Chronic Lymphocytic	18-G	Hyperplasia	18-A,B,C,D,E,H(1)
Chronic Myelocytic	18-H	Normal	16-4;18-A1,F1
Erythroblast	16-19;18-E24	Replaced by Leukemic Tissue	18-G1,H1,I1
Endothelial	17-C2	BONES	
Erythroblastosis Fetalis	18-E18 to E 24	Bones	1;21
Hemohistioblast (stem cell)	16-1;18-I12	Acromion	1-12;19-107;21-24
Lead Poisoning	18-E6 to E12	Asterion	21-7
Leukocytes	17-C1,E2,C3	Atlas	21-13
Lymphoblast	16-7;18-G12	Axis	21-14
Lymphocyte	16-25;17-NBC,18-G13,I13	Bregma	19-3
Megakaryocyte	16-12	Calcaneus	19-71;21-47
Megaloblast	18-B10	Capitate	19-46;21-33
Metamyelocyte		Carpals	1-33
Basophilic	16-16	Clavicle	1-10;19-110;21-21;26-34
Eosinophilic	16-15;18-H17	Coccyx	1-29;21-20
Neutrophilic	16-14;18-H16	Coracoid Process	1-13;19-109
Monoblast	16-3	Coronoid Process	19-14
Monocyte	16-24;18-A10,F7	Cuboid	19-78;21-48
Myeloblast	16-2;18-H11	Cuneiform	
Basophilic	16-11;18-H14	First	19-76;21-51
Eosinophilic	16-10;18-H15	Second	19-69;21-50
Neutrophilic	16-9;18-H12,H13	Third	19-68;21-49
Normoblast	16-13;18-E15,E23,I11	Femur	1-36;19-83'21-41
Neutrophil	18-A7,B11,C10,D11,F10	Head of	1-30;19-57
Platelet	16-20;17-E2;18-A11 B13,C12,D14,E12,E17,F11, G14,H21,I14	Neck of	19-58;21-42
		Fibula	1-40;19-80;21-46
Proerythroblast	16-8	Frontal	1-1;14-2,30;19-6
Polychromatophilia	18-D7,E7,E14,E22,G10,H10,I10	Frontal Process	14-19
Red		Glabella	19-8
Adult	16-19	Hamate	19-49;21-34
Carbon Dioxide Release	17-A3,A5,A6	Humerus	1-17;19-104;21-25;26-24
Diseased		Condyle of	1-21
Macrocyte	18-B6,E18	Head of	1-14
Microcyte	18-C6,D6	Hyoid	5-10;19-17;20-III13
Stippled	18-E6	Ilium	19-55;21-38
Exchange of Oxygen and		Iliac Crest	1-22;10-D17;17-D;21-39
Carbon Dioxide	17-A3	Iliac Fossa	1-23
Function	17-A	Iliac Spine, Anterior Superior	1-25
Macrocytic	18-B2	Inion	19-121;21-3
Microcytic	18-C2	Ischium	1-32;19-87;21-40
Normal	17-NBC; 18-A2,A6,F2,F6 G2,G6; I-26,I-6	Lacrimal	19-12
		Lambda	19-124;21-8
Normal Volume	17-E; 18-A3	Lateral Epicondyle	1-38
Normocytic	18-D2,E2	Lateral Malleolus	1-42
Oxygen enters	17-A3,A7,A8	Lunate	19-50;21-29
Regeneration		Malar:See Zygomatic Bone	19-13
Decreased	18-B2,C2	Mandible	1-8;5-11;19-16, 20-III16,IIB20
Increased	18-E2,G2,H2,I2	Ascending Ramus of	21-6
Normal	18-A2	Manubrium of Sternum	1-11;19-23
		Mastoid Process	9-A7;21-5
		Maxilla	1-7;14-11;19-15

Anatomical Feature	Chart number, bold Feature number, light	Anatomical Feature	Chart number, bold Feature number, light
BONES (Continued)		**BRAIN (Continued)**	
Nasal Process of	**15**-30	Cortical Area of Larynx	**26**-50
Medial Epicondyle	**1**-37	Eyes, Conjugated Movement	**26**-55
Medial Malleolus	**1**-46	Fingers, Function of	**26**-54
Metacarpals	**1**-34;**19**-85;**21**-36	Functional Areas of Brain	
Metatarsals	**1**-44;**19**-77;**21**-52	Auditory Speech Area	**26**-11
Nasal	**1**-5;**14**-27;**15**-29;**19**-11	Ankle	**26**-59
Nasion	**19**-10	Conjugated Movements of Eyes	**26**-55
Navicular	**19**-75	Cortical Area of Larynx	**26**-50
Obelion	**19**-125	Fingers	**26**-54
Occipital	**19**-123;**21**-2	Hearing	**26**-10
Ophryon	**19**-7	Hip	**26**-58
Parietal	**1**-2;**19**-126;**21**-1	Motor Speech Area	**26**-48
Patella	**1**-39;**19**-82	Mouth	**26**-52
Phalanges	**1**-35,45;**19**-84,70;**21**-37,53	Muscle Sensation	**26**-5
Pisiform	**19**-48;**21**-35	Post Central Gyrus	
Pterion	**19**-5	(Sensory Area)	**26**-2
Pubis	**19**-56	Shoulder	**26**-57
Pubic Symphysis	**1**-31;**12**-A9;**13**-A7;**19**-89	Smell	**26**-45
Radius	**1**-27;**19**-95;**21**-27	Taste	**26**-46
Ribs	**21**-17	Tongue	**26**-51
Cross Section	**16**-4	Vision	**26**-12
Eleventh Thoracic	**10**-D23	Visual Speech Area	**26**-9
First	**26**-33	Wrist	**26**-56
Twelfth	**1**-20	Writing	**26**-7
Sacrum	**1**-28;**21**-19	Gray Matter	**15**-5;**27**-C8
Scaphoid	**19**-40;**21**-28	Hearing, Function of	**26**-10
Scapula	**1**-15;**19**-24;**21**-22;**26**-25	Hip, Function of	**26**-58
Spine of	**21**-21	Horizontal Section	**27**-B
Skull	**15**-6;**26**-4	Lobe	
Sphenoid	**1**-3;**19**-9	Frontal	**26**-53
Stephanion	**19**-4	Occipital	**26**-13
Sternum	**16**-4	Parietal	**26**-6
Body of	**1**-16 **19**-29;**26**-30	Temporal	**26**-14
Manubrium of	**1**-11	Median Sagittal Section	**27**-D
Styloid Process	**9**-A8	Mid-Brain	**15**-15;**26**-15;**30**-B1
Talus	**19**-79	Motor Speech Area	**26**-48
Tarsals	**1**-43	Mouth, Function of	**26**-52
Temporal	**1**-4;**9**-A32;**19**-2;**21**-4	Muscle Sensation Area	**26**-5
Inferior Line	**19**-1	Pole	
Mastoid process of	**9**-A7;**21**-5	Frontal	**27**-D19,B5,A1
Petrous Part of	**9**-A25	Occipital	**27**-D39,B13
Styloid Process of	**9**-A8	Temporal	**27**-A8
Superior Line	**19**-127	Pre-Central Gyrus	
Tibia	**1**-41;**19**-81;**21**-45	(Motor Area)	**26**-1
Trapezium	**19**-41;**21**-31	Section, Horizontal	**27**-B
Trapezoid	**19**-42;**21**-32	Sensory Cortex	**27**-D8
Triquetrum	**19**-47;**21**-30	Shoulder, Function of	**26**-57
Trochanter		Sight as a function of Brain	**15**
Greater	**19**-59;**21**-43	Smell, Function of	**26**-45
Lesser	**19**-60;**21**-44	Sulcus, Central	**26**-3
Ulna	**1**-26;**19**-96;**21**-26	Sylvian Fissure	**26**-49
Vertebra		Taste, Function of	**26**-46
Cervical	**1**-9;**21**-15	Tela Choroidea of Third Ventricle	**27**-D12
Lumbar	**21**-18	Tongue, Function of	**26**-51
Fifth Lumbar	**1**-24	Uncus	**27**-A27
Thoracic	**21**-16	Ventricle, Fourth	**15**-10;**27**-D35
Twelfth Thoracic	**1**-19	Lateral, Anterior Horn	**27**-B2
Vertebral Column	**26**-23	Inferior Horn	**27**-B19
Vertex	**19**-128;**21**-9	Posterior Horn	**27**-B15
Xiphoid Process	**1**-18	Third	**27**-D10,B21
Zygomatic Arch	**1**-6;**14**-10;**26**-43	Vision, Function of	**26**-12
Zygomatic (Malar)	**15**-I	Visual Speech Area	**26**-9
Bowman's Capsule	**10**-C1B	White Matter	**27**-C7
Brachial Plexus	**21**-88	Wrist, Function of	**26**-56
		Writing, Function of	**26**-7
BRAIN		Branchial Arches	**11**-K2
Brain	**15**-7; **26**;**27**	Breathing, Position of Larynx	
Ankle, Function of	**26**-59	and Pharynx in	**20**-IIB
Anterior Commissure	**27**-D32	Bregma	**19**-3
Auditory Speech Area	**26**-11	Bronchioles	**7**-17
Base of Brain	**27**-A	Bronchitis, Acute Tracheo	**8**-E
Anterior Perforated Surface	**27**-A30	**BRONCHUS (BRONCHI)**	
Callosal Sulcus	**27**-D16	Inflamed, Cross Section	**8**-E
Caudate Nucleus	**27**-B6	Left Main	**5**-14;**7**-13
Centrum Semiovale		Ramification	**7**-17
(White Matter)	**15**-7		
Cerebellum	**26**-17;**27**-A-16;**27**-D36	**C**	
Cerebrum	**21**-101	Calcaneus	**19**-71;**21**-47
Cingulate Gyrus	**27**-D7,D17	Calcar Avis	**27**-B16
Cingulate Sulcus	**27**-D14	Candida Albicans	**20**-IVB
Cortex of	**2**-2	Capitate Bone	**19**-46;**21**-33
		CANAL	
		Central, of Spinal Cord	**27**-C6,D32

Anatomical Feature	Chart number, bold Feature number, light	Anatomical Feature	Chart number, bold Feature number, light
CANAL (Continued)		COLON	
Lateral, of Ear	9-B12	Ascending	5-39;19-92;21-107;25-J13
Posterior, of Ear	9-B1	Descending	5-29;19-54;21-108
Semicircular, of Ear	9-A28	Distal	30-E11
Cardiac Opening of Stomach	5-16	Hepatic Flexure	5-40
CAPILLARIES		Lymph Nodes and Vessels	25-J
Alveolar	17-A9	Sigmoid	5-32;13-A2
Alveolus and Capillary Network	17-A1	Teniae Coli	5-38
Arterial	17-B4	Transverse	5-27;19-53;25-J6
Lymph Node	24-E	Commissure, Anterior	27-B7
Microscopic Section of Inflamed	17-C	Conchae, Nasal Cavity	
Venous	17-B5	Inferior ,Middle, Superior	7-35;8-A3
Capsule, Bowman's	10-C16	Conjunctiva	2-22
Capsule, Renal	10-A1	Connective Tissue	29
Carpals	1-33	Coracoid Process of Scapula	1-13;19-109
CARTILAGE		CORD	
Costal	19-28	Spermatic	13-A19,B14
Cricoid	20-IIB12,III8	Spinal: see Spinal Cord	
Ear	9-A2,6,13, 15	Umbilical	11-H-7,K5;12-C6
Elastic	29-9	Vocal: see Vocal Cord	
Fibrocartilage	29-10	Corium, Skin	3-III
Hyaline	29-8	Cornea	2-27
Hyoid Bone with	20-III13,IIB17	Coronoid Process of Mandible	19-14
Nasal, Lateral	14-18	Corpuscles of Ruffini	3-15
Thyroid	19-18;20-IIB16,III6	Corpus Callosum	7-2;27-D18,B4
Horn of		Corpus Cavernosum	13-A12
Superior	20-IIB9,III12	Corpus Spongiosum	13-A11
Inferior	20-IIB11,III11	CORTEX	
Caudate Nucleus	27-B6	of Adrenal Glands	23-4 b
CAVITY		of Brain	2-2
Oral	5-1;8-A4	Cortex	10-C15
Cross Section	25-H7	Gray	15-5
Nasal (Conchae)	5-2; 7-35;20-B22;25-H8	of Hair	3-2
Cross Section	8-B7	of Kidneys	10-A2
CECUM		Motor, Brain	27-D11
Cecum	25-J11	Renal	10-D2
Opened	5-36	Sensory, Brain	27-D8
CELLS		Cuboid Bone	19-78;21-48
Autonomic Ganglion	28-C6	Cuneus	27-D2
Cardiac Muscle	28-B5	CUNEIFORM	
Blood: see Blood Cells		First	19-76;21-51
Division of	11-A-E	Second	19-69;21-50
Endothelial	17-C2	Third	19-68;21-49
Ethmoid, Air	8-B13;15-31	Cupula, Ear	9-B7
Purkinje	28-C5		
Pyramidal	28-C4		
Skeletal Muscle	28-B1	**D**	
Sickle Shaped, red blood	18-E13	Deltoid	21-55
Smooth Muscle	28-B3	Development of the Blood Cell	16
CEREBELLUM		Development of the Embryo	11
Cerebellum	7-4;26-17;27-D36,A-16	DIAPHRAGM	
Peduncle		Diaphragm	5-18;7-19;8-A8; 10-D26; 26-27
Superior	15-13	Urogenital	13-A21
Middle	15-14	DIGESTIVE SYSTEM	
Vermis of	27-B14	Digestive System	5
CEREBRUM		Disorders of	6
Cerebrum	21-101	Diphtheria (Pharyngeal Group)	20-IVC
Cerebral Peduncle	27-A10 ,B16	Diseases of the Blood Cells	18
Precuneus	27-D6	DUCTS	
Cervical Lymph Nodes	24-A3,A32	Bile	6-A4;30-E8
Cervical Nerves	21-83	Common, Ear	9-B11
Cervical Vertebrae	1-9;21-15	Cystic	6-A3
Cervix	11-J14;12-A17	Efferent	13-B10
Chest, Sagittal	8-A;26	Ejaculatory	13-A23
Chordae Tendineae	4-A18	Hepatic	5-44;6-A2
Choroid	2-16	Lacrimal (Tear)	14-3,24, 25, 28
Chorion	11-H4	Lateral	9-B12
Chyliferous Plexus	25-G2	Lymph, filled with Chyle	6-C6
Chyle System in Small Intestine	25-G	Lymphatic, Right	24-A30
Circulation of Blood	19	Nasolacrimal	14-17
Cisterna Chyli	24-A12	Opening of	14-16
Clavicle	1-10;19-110;21-21;26-34	Pancreatic	6-A5
Coccyx	1-29;21-20	Parotid	26-40
COCHLEA		Superior	9-B10
Cochlea	9-A17	Thoracic	24-A8
Apical Spiral	9-B5	End of	24-A4
Cupula	9-B7	Vas Deferens	13-A9,B16
Fenestra of	9-A11	Duodenum	5-41;6-A7;25-J14,K7
Middle Spiral	9-B6		
Modiolus	9-A20		
Nerve	9-A22	**E**	
Coelom ,Extra Embryonic	11-H1	EAR	
Collateral Eminence, Brain	27-B11	Development of, in Embryo	11-K1
Colliculi, Superior & Inferior	27-B12	External Acoustic Meatus	9-A3
		External Ear (Aurical)	9-A1,A33

Anatomical Feature	Chart number, bold Feature number, light
EAR (continued)	
Glands (Cerumen)	9-A5
Hairs	9-A4
Hearing, Functional Area of Brain	26-10
Inner (Labyrinth)	9-A35
Malleus	9-A31
Middle	9-A10,A34
Middle Spiral	9-B6
Modiolus	9-A20
Osseous Spiral	9-18
Sectioned Vertically	
Spiral Lamina	9A
Tympanic Membrane	9-A18
Window	9-A9
Oval	9-A27,B4
Round	9-A12,B3
Efferent Lymph Vessels	24-D2
Elastic Cartilage Tissue	29-9
Elastic Tissue	29-6
EMBRYO, HUMAN	
Cells and Cell Division	11
Development of	
Eighth Week	11-L
Fifth Week	11-K
Heart	11-K7
Human Egg	
Fertilized	11-A,B,C,D,E
Embedding in Endometrium	11-J9
Germinal Spot	11-G3
Surrounded by Sperms	11-G
Yolk	11-H8
Mesenchymal Tissue	29-1
Pregnancy at Term	12-B
Third Week	11-H
Uterus, Fallopian Tubes, Ovaries	11-J
ENDOCRINE GLANDS	22
Diagram of Interrelations	23
Eosinophils	
Normal Quantity	17-NBC
See also Blood Cells	
Epidermis	3-II
Epididymis	13-A18,B9,B13
Epiglotis	5-9;7-28;20-IB2,IIB7,III4
Aryepiglottic Fold	20-IB11
Tubercle of	20-IA2,IB2
Epithelial Tissue	28-A
Erythroblast	18-E24
Erythroblastosis Fetalis	18-E18 to 24
Erythrocytes: see Blood Cells, Red	
ESOPHAGUS	
Esophagus	5-13;10-D1;19-31
Cross Section through	6-D1
Opening of	7-10
Eustachian Tube	9-A14
Orifice of	7-34
External Acoustic Meatus	9-A3
EYE	2; 14; 15
Anterior Chamber	2-28
Autonomic Nervous System	30-E1
Choroid	2-16
Ciliary Muscle	2-18
Conjunctiva	2-22
Cornea	2-27
in Embryo	11-K8
Eyeball	14-7
Periorbital Fat	2-13;15-35
Fornix of Conjunctiva	2-21,30
Fovea	2-6
Frontal Section	8-B3
Functional Area of Brain	
Conjugated movement of Eyes	26-55
Iris	2-25;14-6
Lacrimal	
Canals	14-24,28
Caruncle	14-23
Glands	14-3;15-21;26-44;30-E2
Sac	14-25;15-27
Lens	2-34
Optic Chiasma	15-33;27-D25,A4
Optic Tract	15-19;27-A7
Orbicularis Oculi	15-36;26-42
Orbital Wall	2-33
Posterior Chamber	2-24

Anatomical Feature	Chart number, bold Feature number, light
EYE (continued)	
Protective Mechanism	14
Pupil	14-5
Retina,	
Nasal	15-32
Temporal	15-38;2-12
Sclera	2-17
Sight as a Function of Brain	15
Vitreous Body	2-11
See also Vision	
F	
Fallopian Tubes	11-J
Isthmus	11-J2
Ampulla	11-J4
Female Reproductive Organs	12
FEMUR	1-36;19-83;21-41
Head of	1-30
Neck of	19-58; 21-42
Fenestra	
Vestibular	9-A11;B-8
FIBERS	
Para Sympathetic	30
Sympathetic	30
Sympathetic Chain	30-A
Fibrocartilage	29-10
Fibrous Tissue	29-7
Fibula	1-40;19-80;21-46
Fimbria	11-J6
Flocculus	27-A12
FORNIX	
Fornix	27-D20
Columns of	27-B1
of Conjunctiva	2-21,30
of Vagina	11-J11
Frontal Bone	1-1;14-2,30;19-6
Frontal Process	14-19
Fundus of Uterus	12-A4
G	
Gall Bladder	5-45;19-99;25-J18;30-E8
Gallstones	6-A1
GANGLION	
Autonomic	28-C6
Celiac	30-D5
Ciliary	30-D1
Dorsal Root	27-C11
Gasserion	19-122
Mesenteric	
Inferior	30-D7
Superior	30-D6
Otic	30-D3
Sphenopalatine	8-D7;30-D2
Submandibular	30-D4
Germinal Disc	11-F1
Germinal Spot	11-G3
Germinal Vesicle	11-G2
Glabella	19-8
GLANDS	
Adrenal	10-D3,D24;21-105;22-5;23-4
Cortex of	23-4b
Medulla of	23-4a
Bulbo-urethral	13-A20
Ear, Glands (Cerumen)	9-A5
Endocrine	22
Diagram of Interrelations	23
Lacrimal	14-3;15-21;26-44;30-E2
Lymph: see Lymph Nodes	
Parathyroid	23-7a
Parotid	19120;26-39;30-E3
Pineal	22-1;23-1;27-D5,B9
Pituitary	7-1;22-2;23-2;27-A31
Anterior	23-2b;27-D27
Posteior	23-2a;27-D28
Prostate	13-A22,B7
Sebaceous	3-I12
Sublingual	30-E4
Submaxillary	20-III14;30-E4
Sudoriferous (Sweat),	24-F4
Duct of Sweat Gland	3-I6;24-F7
Spherical Body of	3-I14
Suprarenal, Right and Left	10-D3,D24;21-105
Tarsal	2-29;14-4,12

Anatomical Feature	Chart number, bold Feature number, light
GLANDS (Continued)	
Thymus	**22**-4;**23**-6;**26**-31
Thyroid	**20**-IIB14,III10;**22**-3;**23**-3;**26**-36
Glans Penis	**13**-A14
Glomerulus in Kidney	**10**-C1a
GONADS	**23**-7
Ovary	**11**-J19,J8;**12**-A3;**22**-7;**23**-7b
Testis	**13**-A17,B12;**23**-7a
Gray Matter	**27**-C8
GYRUS	
Hippocampal, Uncus of	**27**-B18
Post Central	**26**-2
Pre Central	**26**-1
H	
HAIR	
Bulb of	**3**-24
Cortex	**3**-2
Cuticle	**3**-3
in Ear	**9**-A4
Follicle	**24**-F1
Medulla of	**3**-1
Papilla	**3**-23
Root of	**3**-22;**25**
Dermic Coat	**3**-20
Epidermic Coat	**3**-21
Shaft of	**3**-I
HEAD	
Frontal Section of	**8**-B
Head Cold with Sinusitis, Symptoms of Common	**8**-D
Sagittal Section of	**8**-A;**26**-E
HEART	
Heart	**1**-56;**4**;**19**-30;**26**-28;**30**-E5
Anterior View	**4**-D
Apex	**4**-A21
Atrium	
Left	**4**-A12,C4,D5
Right	**4**-A29,B4,C6
Cardiac Tissue	**28**-B5
Coronary Sinus	**4**-B7
Cross Section	**4**-C
Fat of	**4**-B10,D9
Muscular Interventricular Septum	**4**-A26
Anterior Sulcus	**4**-D7
Posterior Sulcus	**4**-B9
Myocardium	**4**-A17,23
Nervous System and	**26E**
Posterior View	**4**-B
Ventricle	
Left	**4**-A15,B8
Right	**4**-A28,D8;**7**-20
Haustra	**5**-37
Hematocrit Tube	**17**-E
Hemoglobin	**17**-NBC
Hemohistioblast	**16**-1
Henle's Loop	**10**-C11
Hilum of Kidney	**10**-D5
Hilius of Lymphnode	**24**-B6,B8
Hippocampus	**27**-B10
Fimbria of	**27**-B17
Hippocampal Digitations	**27**-B20
Uncus of Hippocampal Gyrus	**27**-B18
HUMAN BODY	
Back View with Bones, Muscles, Nerves, Viscera	**21**
Front View	**19**
Bones and Arteries	**1**
Digestive System	**5**
Endocrine System	**22**
Lymphatic System	**24**-A
Organs and Cirulation	**19**
Humerus	**1**-21;**19**-104;**21**-25;**26**-24
Condyle of	**1**-21
Head of	**1**-14
Hyaline Cartilage Tissue	**29**-8
Hyperopia	**2**-C
Hypogastric Lymph Nodes	**24**-A14
I	
ILIUM	**19**-55;**21**-38

Anatomical Feature	Chart number, bold Feature number, light
ILIUM (Continued)	
Iliac Crest	**1**-22;**10**-D17;**21**-39
Iliac Fossa	**1**-23
Iliac Lymph Nodes, External	**24**-A20
Incus	**9**-30
Infundibulum	**27**-D26,A6
Inguinal Lymph Nodes	**24**-A19
Inguinal Vessels and Lymph Nodes	**24**-A16
Intercostal Nerves to Intercostal and Abdominal Muscles	**8**-A10
Intertubercular Sulcus	**19**-106
Interventricular Foramen	**27**-D22
Intestinal Villus and Digestive Disorders	**6**
INTESTINES	**30**-E10
Large: see Colon	
Lymph Nodes and Vessels of	**25**-K
Microscopic Section with Chyle System	**25**-G
Small	**6**;**5**-30;**19**-97;**25**-K5
Iris	**2**-25;**14**-6
Ischium	**1**-32;**19**-87;**21**-40
J	
Jejunum	**5**-28
K	
KIDNEYS	
Kidneys	**10**;**19**-51;**21**-106;**30**-E9
Alcoholic	**10**-B2
Calcyes	
Major	**10**-A8
Minor	**10**-A9
Capsule	**10**-A1
Cortex of	**10**-A2;**10**-C15
Distal Convoluted Tubule	**10**-C8
Disorders	**10**-B
Hilum of	**10**-D5
Inner Zone	**10**-C13
Interlobular Artery	**10**-C6
Interlobular Vein	**10**-C7
Left (Section)	**10**-D4
Location of	**10**-D
Longitudinal Section	**10**-A
Medulla	**10**-A3,C16
Nephron	**10**-A4
Outer Zone	**10**-C14
Pelvis of	**10**-A11,D6
Pyelonephritis (Cross Section)	**10**-B3
Pyramids	**10**-A7,D7
Papilla	**10**-A15
Ramification of Arteries	**10**-A5
Ramification of Veins	**10**-A6
Right	**10**-D19
Staghorn Calculus	**10**-B1
Stone in	**10**-B1
Renal Corpuscle	**10**-C1
Renal Sinus	**10**-A14
L	
Labyrinth (Inner Ear)	**9**-35
Labia Majora	**12**-A14
Labia Minora	**12**-A13
Lacrimal Gland	**14**-3;**15**-21;**26**-44;**30**-E2
Lacus Lacrimalus	**14**-22
Lambda	**19**-124;**21**-8
Lacteal	**6**-C2;**25**-G1,I1
LAMINA	
Spiral	**9**-18
Superior & Inferior Colliculli	**27**-D37
Terminalis	**27**-D24
Large Intestine: see Colon	
LARYNX	
Larynx	**7**-27;**8**-A5;**20**,**25**-H5;**26**-37
Cortical Area of	**26**-50
Entrance to	**20**-IIB8
From above	**20**-IA,IB
Frontal Section	**20**-III
Laryngeal Polyp	**20**-IC1
Piriform Recess	**20**-IA6,IB6
Position in Breathing	**5**-49;**20**-IIB
Position in Swallowing	**5**-50;**20**-IIA
Laryngopharynx	**7**-9;**8**-A12

Anatomical Feature	Chart number, bold Feature number, light
Lateral Duct	**9**-B12
Lead Poisoning	**18**-E6 to E12
Lens	**15**-37
LEUCOCYTE: see Blood Cells, White	
LEUKEMIA	
Acute	**18**-I
Lymphatic, Chronic	**18**-G
Myelocytic, Chronic	**18**-H
LIGAMENTS	
Arteriosum	**4**-A10,B13
Broad, of Uterus	**11**-J17
Cricothyroid	**20**-IIB15,III7
Palpebral	
Lateral	**14**-8
Medial	**14**-26
Round, of Uterus	**11**-J18;**12**-A6
Ovarian	**11**-J22
Suspensory, of Crystalline Lens	**2**-35
Sacrouterine	**12**-A19
LIMBS	
Lower	**11**-K4
Upper	**11**-K6
LIVER	
Liver	**19**-101;**25**-J17;**30**-E8
Diseased	**6**-A8
Healthy	**5**-42,46
Lymph Nodes and Vessels	**25**-J
LOBE	
Frontal, of Brain	**26**-53
Hypophysis	**27**-D27,D28
Lung	**7**-16,24
Occipital	**26**-13
Parietal	**26**-6
Temporal	**26**-14
Lumbar Vertebrae	**1**-24;**21**-18
LUNGS	**21**-102;**30**-E6
Alveolar Sacs (Magnified View)	**7**-14
Alveolus (Magnified View)	**7**-15
Left	**4**-A9;**5**-15;**19**-25;**26**-29
Apex of	**7**-12
Cross Section of	**7**-16
Right	**4**-A1;**5**-48;**7**-24;**19**-108
Vessels and Lymph Nodes	**24**-A7
LYMPHATIC SYSTEM	**24**;**25**
LYMPH NODES	
Aortic, Lateral	**24**-A23
Auricular, Posterior	**24**-A1
Axillary	**24**-A5,26
Buccal	**24**-A35
Capillaries	**6**-C2;**24**-C
Capsule	**25**-B5
Celiac	**25**-K10
Cervical	**24**-A3,A32
Superior, Deep	**24**-A32
Colic, Right	**25**-J12
Cross Section	**16**-6;**24**-B
Follicle with Germinal Center	**24**-B4
Gastric	
Superior	**25**-J4
Interior	**25**-J5
Hepatic	**25**-J19
Hypogastric	**24**-A14
Iliac	
Common	**24**-A21
External	**24**-A20
Inguinal	**24**-A16,A19
Magnified	**24**-B
Mandibular	**24**-A33
Maxillary	**24**-A36
Medullary Sinus	**24**-B7
Mesenteric	**25**-K6
Mesocolic	**25**-J7
Nodule	**6**-C5
Cortical	**24**-B3
Occipital	**24**-A2
Pancreaticolienal	**25**-K3,J2
Paracardial	**25**-J1
Parotid	**24**-37
Pleura and Lung	**24**-A7
Sacral	**24**-A15
Splenic	**25**-K2
Subclavicular	**24**-A28
Subinguinal	**24**-A18
Submental	**24**-A34
Subpyloric	**25**-K9
LYMPH NODES (Continued)	
Superficial	**24**-A24
Supratrochlear	**24**-A22
Trabecula	**24**-B2
Tracheal	**24**-A31
Lymphoblast	**16**-7; **18**-G12
LYMPHOCYTE	**17**-NBC; **18**-A9,B12,C11,D13 F9,G13,I13
Atypical	**18**-F8
Large	**16**-25
Small	**16**-17
LYMPH VESSELS	**24**-F2; **25**
Afferent	**24**-B1,E1
Chyliferous	**25**-G2
Cisterna Chyli	**24**-A12
Cross Section	**24**-F
Efferent	**24**-B6,E2
Ileocolic Chain	**25**-J9
Inguinal	**24**-A16
Lumbar Chain	**24**-A13
Mediastinal	**24**-A27
Paracolic Chain	**25**-J8
Parotid	**24**-A37
of Pleura and Lung	**24**-A7
Intercostal	**24**-A9
Renal	**24**-A11
of Skin	**24**-F
of Small Intestines	**25**-K
Supra Trochlear	
Splenic	**24**-A10
of Stomach, Liver, and Large Intestines	**25**-J
Subpyloric	**25**-J15
M	
Macrocyte	**18**-B6, E18
Male Reproductive Organs	**13**
Malleus	**9**-A3
Mamillary Body	**27**-A29,D29
Mandible	**1**-8;**19**-16
Ascending Ramus of	**21**-6
Manubrium	**1**-11; **19**-23
Massa Intermedia	**27**-B8,D13
Mastoid Process	**9**-A7;**21**-5
MATTER	
Gray	**27**-C8
White	**27**-C7
Median Sagital Section of Brain	**27**
MEDULLA	
of Adrenal Gland	**23**-4a
of Hair	**3**-1
of Kidney	**10**-A3,
Oblongata	**7**-6;**26**-19;**27**-D31,A18;**30**-B2
Spinalis	**7**-8
Pyramids	**10**-D7
Inner Zone	**10**-C13
Outer Zone	**10**-C14
Megakaryocyte	**16**-12
Megaloblast	**18**-B10
MEMBRANE	
Development in Embryo	**11**-H
Mucous	
Inflammatory Hyperemia	**8**-D2
Inflammatory Vascular Dilitation	**8**-E1
Thyrohyoid	**20**-III5
Mesosalpinx	**11**-J21
Mesentery	**6**-B
Metacarpals	**1**-34
Metamyelocyte	
Basophilic	**16**-16
Eosinophilic	**16**-15;**18**-H17
Neutrophilic	**16**-14;**18**-H16
Metatarsals	**1**-44;**19**-77;**21**-52
Microcyte	**18**-C6,D6
Mid-Brain	**15**-15;**26**-15;**30**-B1
Modiolus	**9**-A20
Monoblast	**16**-3
Monocyte	**16**-24;**17**-NBC;**18**-A10,F7
Mononucleosis, Infectious	**18**-F
MOUTH	

Anatomical Feature	Chart number, bold Feature number, light	Anatomical Feature	Chart number, bold Feature number, light
MOUTH (Continued)		NERVES (Continued)	
Mouth, Functional	26-52	Cervical	21-83
Frontal Section through	20-III	Cervical Plexus	21-87
MUSCLES		Cochlear	9-22
Muscles	21	Cross Section of	3-18
Adductor Magnus	21-72	Facial (VII)	27-A24
Arrector Pili	3-13	Glossopharyngeal (IX)	27-A20
Biceps Femoris	21-70	Hypoglossal (XII)	27-A14
Brachialis	21-57	Infraorbital Foramen	14-15
Brachioradialis	21-58	Intercostal	8-A10
Ciliary	2-19	Intermediate Nerve	27-A22
Deltoid	21-55	Lateral Femoral Cutaneous	21-96
Dorsal Interossei (hand)	21-62	Lumbar	21-85
Extensor Carpi Radialis	21-60	Medial Brachial Cutaneous	21-95
Extensor Carpi Ulnaris	21-61	Median	21-90
Extensor Digitorum	21-59	Motor	27-C12
Flexor Digitorum Longus	21-81	Nervous Control of Respiration	8
Gastrocnemius	21-78	Oculomotor (III)	27-A28,D34
Geniohyoid	5-7; 20-IIB19	Optic (II)	2-10;15-20,34;27-A5
Glossopalatine	20-III1	Olfactory	
Gluteus Maximus	21-69	Bulb (I)	27-A2
Gluteus Medius	21-66	Tract (I)	27-A3
Gracilis	21-75	with Intranasal Ramifications	8-D1
of Heart	4-A26,17,23	Peroneal, Common	21-99
Iliacus	10-D16	Pelvic	30-C5
Interossei, Dorsal	21-62	Phrenic	7-11;8-A11
Interventricular	4-A26	Left	7-18
Latissimus Dorsi	21-65	Right	7-21
Levator Palpebrae Superioris	15-24;2-3,31	Posterior Brachial Cutaneous	21-91
Mastication	26-38	Posterior Femoral Cutaneous	21-97
Muscular Tissue	28-B	Radial	21-89
Mylohyoid	5-8; 20-IIB18	Deep Branch of Radial	21-92,93
Oblique, External	21-68	Sacral	21-86
Inferior (Eye)	2-15;14-14;15-22	Sciatic	21-98
Superior (Eye)	2-4;14-31;15-26	Sensory	
Opponens Digiti Minimi	21-63	of Skin	3-5
Orbicularis Oculi	2-20,32;15-36	with Dorsal Root Ganglion	27-C11
Papillary	4-A19	Spermatic Cord	13-A19,B14
Peroneus Longus	21-80	Splanchnic	30-C2,C3,C4
Psoas Major	10-D15	Thoracic	21-84
Rectus, of Eye		Tibial	21-100
Inferior	2-14;14-13	Trigeminal (V)	8-D6;27-A23
Lateral	14-9;15-23	Trochlear (IV)	27-A25
Medialis	14-29;15-25	Ulnar	21-94
Superior	2-5;14-1;15-24	Vagus	8-A1;26-21;27-A13;30-C1
Sartorius	21-76	to Larynx, Lung and Aorta, Heart	8-A1
Semimembranosus	21-73	Vestibular	9-24
Semitendinous	21-74	Vestibulocochlear (VII)	27-A21
Septim (Interventricular)	4-A26	Nervous Control of Respiration	
Soleus	21-79	and Symptoms of Infections	8
Sternocleidomastoid	21-54	Nervous System and Heart	28-C
of Stomach	6-D6	Neurons	28-C
Temporal	15-4	Types of	
Tendon Calcanean	21-82	Neutrophils	17-NBC
Tensor Fasciae Latae	21-67	Normal Quantity	
Tensor Tympani	9-A29	Mature	16-21
Teres Major	21-64	NODES: See Lymph Nodes	
Triceps	21-56	Normoblast	16-13;18-E15,E23,G11,I11
Vastus Lateralis	21-71	NOSE	
Vastus Medialis	21-77	Meatus	8-B4,B9
Zygomaticus Major	26-41	Nasal Bone	1-5;14-27;15-29;19-11
Muscular Tissue	28-B	Nasal Cartilage	14-18
Myeloblast	16-2	Nasal Cavity	7-35
MYELOCYTE		Cross Section of	8-B5
Basophilic	16-11;18-H14	Nasal Passage	20-IIB22
Eosinophilic	16-10;18-H15	Nasal Septum	8-B12;15-28
Neutrophilic	16-9;18-H12,H13,H18		
Myometrium	11-J15		
Myopia	2-B	**O**	
		Occipital Bone	19-123
		Occipital Lymph Nodes	24-A2
N		Occipital Protuberance	21-3
Nasal Concha	8-B10,B11	Olfactory Bulb	27-A2
Nasal Process	15-30	Olfactory Tract	27-A3
Nasopharynx	7-5;8-A14;20-IIB2	Optic Chiasma	15-33;27-A4,D25
Nasalacrimal Duct	14-17	Optic Papilla	2-9
Neck, Sagittal Section	26	Optic Tract	15-19;27-A7
Nephron	10-A4,C	Oral Cavity	7-32
NERVES		Oropharynx	7-7;8-A13;18-13;20-IIB6
Nerves	21	Ovary (Ovaries)	11-J19;12-A3;22-7;23-7b
Abducens (VI)	27-A11	Follicles	11-J3
Accessory (XI)	27-A15	Opened; Section	11-J8
Auditory	9-23		
Brachial Plexus	21-88		

Anatomical Feature	Chart number, bold Feature number, light
OVARIES (Continued)	
Oviduct	**11**-J5,J20,J7;**12**-A2;**23**
End of	**11**-J7
Ovum, Fertilized, Embedding in Endometrium	**11**-J9
P	
Palate	
Hard Palate	**5**-3; **7**-33; **20**-III17
In Breathing	**5**-49
Soft Palate	**5**-4; **7**-31;**20**-IIB3
In Swallowing	**5**-50
PANCREAS	
Pancreas	**5**-26a,b,c;**19**-52;**22**-6;**23**-5;**25**-K4
Duct	**6**-A5
Papilla, Lacrimal	**14**-21
Parathyroids	**23**-3a
Parietal Bone	**1**-2;**19**-126;**21**-1
Parieto-Occipital Sulcus	**27**-D3
Maxillary Lymphnodes and Vessels	**24**-A36
Parotid Gland	**19**-120;**26**-39;**30**-E3
Patella	**1**-39;**19**-82
PEDUNCLE	
Cerebral	**27**-A10
Middle Cerebellar	**15**-14
Superior Cerebellar	**15**-13
Pelvis	
Female, Section	**12**-A
Male, Section	**13**
Pericardium	**4**-A22,B5
Periorbital Fat	**2**-13
Peritoneum	**13**-A5
Phalanges	**1**-35,45;**19**-70,84;**21**-37,53
PHARYNX	
Pharynx	**20**-IIA,IIB4,III3
Cross-Section	**25**-H
Diptheria	**20**-IVC
Oral	**5**-6
Position in Breathing	**20**-IIB
Position in Swallowing	**20**-IIA
Pineal Body	**22**-1;**23**-1;**27**-B9,D5
Piriform Recess	**20**-IA6,IB6
Pisiform Bone	**19**-48;**21**-35
PITUITARY GLAND	**7**-1;**8**-A2;**22**-2;**23**-2
Anterior	**23**-2b;**27**-D27
Posterior	**23**-2a;**27**-D28
Placenta	**12**-C1
PLASMA	
Volume	**17**-E
Increased	**18**-B,C,D,E,G,H,I(5)
Normal	**18**-A5,F5
Platelet	**16**-20;**17**-E,2,NBC;**18**-A11,B13 C12,D14,E12,E17,F11,G14,H21,I14
PLEXUS	
Brachial	**21**-88
Cardiac	**26**-26
Cervical	**21**-87
Choroid	**27**-A19
Chyliferous, Internal	**25**-G2
Esophageal	**26**-26
Hypogastric	**30**
at Lymph Capillaries	**24**-C
Mammary	**24**-A25
Pelvic	**30**
Pulmonary	**26**-26
Renal	**24**-A11
Splenic	**24**-A10
Uterine and Ovarian	**24**-A17
Plica Semilunaris	**14**-20
POLE	
Frontal	**27**-A1,B5,D19
Occipital	**27**-B13,D39
Temporal	**27**-A8
Polychromatophilia	**18**-D7,E7,E14,E22,G10,H10 I10
Pons	**7**-3;**26**-18;**27**-A26,D30
Precuneus	**27**-D6
Pregnancy at Term	**12**-B
Pressure Points for Main Arteries	**1**
PROCESSES	
Acromion	**1**-12;**19**-107;**21**-24
Coracoid	**1**-13;**19**-109
Coronoid	**19**-14
Frontal	**14**-19

Anatomical Feature	Chart number, bold Feature number, light
PROCESSES (Continued)	
Mastoid (of Temporal Bone)	**9**-A7;**21**-5
Nasal, of the Maxilla	**15**-30
Styloid (Round Window)	**9**-A12
Xiphoid	**1**-18;**19**-103
Proximal Convoluted Tubule	**10**-C2
Prostate Gland	**13**-A22,B7
Protective Mechanism of the Eye	**14**
Pubic Symphysis	**1**-31;**12**-A9;**13**-A7;**19**-89
Pupil	**2**-26;**14**-5
Pyloric Antrum	**5**-24
Pylorus	**5**-47;**6**-D4;**25**-J16,K8
Deformed by Carcinoma	**6**-D3
R	
Radial Nerve	**21**-89,92,93
Radius (Bone)	**1**-27;**19**-95;**21**-27
RECTUM	
Rectum	**5**-33;**10**-D14;**13**-A26;**12**-A16
Distal Colon	**30**-E11
Renal Calyces	**10**-A8,A9
Renal Lymph Vessels and Plexus	**24**-A11
Renal Pelvis and Blood Vessels	**10**-D6
Renal Pelvis	**10**-A11,D6
Reproductive System, Female	**12**
Reproductive System, Male	**13**
RESPIRATORY TRACT	
Nervous Control of Respiration	**8**
Respiratory Tract	**7**
Symptoms of Infections	**8**
Reticular Tissue	**29**-3
Reticulocyte	**16**-18
Retina	**2**-12
Rima Glottidis	**20**-IA,10,IB10
Rhomboid Fossa	**15**-11
Medial Eminence	**15**-12
Ribs	**1**-20;**10**-D23;**19**-27; **21**-17;**26**-33
S	
Sacral Lymph Nodes	**24**-A15
Sacral Nerves	**21**-86
Sacrum	**1**-28;**21**-19
Sagittal Section of Head Neck and Chest	**26**
Scala Tympani	**9**-A19
Scala Vestibuli	**9**-A21
Scalp	**26**-8
Scapula	**1**-15;**19**-24;**21**-22;**26**-25
Spine of	**21**-23
Sciatic Nerve	**21**-98
Sclera	**2**-17
Scrotum	**13**-A16
Sebaceous Gland	**3**-12
Seminal Vesicles	**13**-A25,B15
Semicircular Canal	**9**-A28
SEPTUM	
Frontal	**8**-B2
Interventricular	**4**-A26
Lymph Node Septum	
System Drainage	**24**-B8
Nasal	**8**-B12;**15**-28
Pellucidum	**27**-B3,D15
Sickle Shaped Red Blood Cells	**18**-E13
Sight as a Function of the Brain	**15**
See also VISION	
SINUSES	
Frontal	**7**-37;**8**-B1;**25**-H1;**26**-47
Maxillary	**8**-B6
Nasal Suppurative Discharge	**8**-D3
Sinusitus	**8**-D
Sphenoidal	**7**-36
Skeleton	**1**
SKIN	
Skin	**3**;**15**-3
Adipose Tissue, Subcutaneous	**3**-IV
Corium, Reticular Layer	**3**-III
Cross Section of	**3**;**17**-B;**24**-F
Dermis	**24**-F5
Epidermis	**3**-II
Sensory Nerve of	**3**-5
Stratum	
Corneum	**3**-7
Granulosum	**3**-9

Anatomical Feature	Chart number, bold Feature number, light
SKIN (Continued)	
Germinativum	3-11
Lucidum	3-8
Spinosum	3-10
Tactile Response	3-A to G
Smell, Functional Area of Brain	26-45
Somites	11-K3
Sperm, Zygote Surrounded by	11-G
Spermatic Cord	13-A19,B14
Sphenoid	1-3;19-9
Spinal Cord	8-A9; 26-22;27-A17,D33
Autonomic Nervous System	30
Central Canal of	27-C6,D32
Cervical Segment of	30-B3
Frontal View, Dura Removed	27-C
Funiculus	27-C2,C4,C4
Horns of, Ventral	27-C9
Dorsal	27-C10
Lumbar Segment	30-B5
Medula Spinalus	7-8
Root of	27-C13,C14
Sacral Segment	30-B6
Thoracic Segment	30-B4
SPLEEN	
Spleen	5-21;21-104;25-K1
Cross Section of	16-5
Lymph Nodes	25-K2
Lymph Vessels and Plexus	24-A10
Splenic Flexure	5-25
Stapes, of Ear	9-A11
STERNUM	1-16;26-30
Body of	19-29
Cross Section of	16-1
Manubrium of	1-11;19-23
STOMACH	
Stomach	5-19;19-33;25-J3;30-E7
Body of	5-20
Diseased	6-D
Fundus	5-17
Lymph Nodes and Vessels	25-J
Movements of During Digestion	6-E7,E2
Mucous Coat	6-D7
Styloid Process	9-A8
Sublingual Gland	30-E4
Submaxillary Gland	20-III14;30-E4
Sweat Gland	3-6,14
SULCUS	
Calcarine Sulcus	27-D1
Central, of Brain	26-3;27-D9
Dorsal Median	27-C5
Longitudinal, of Rhomboid Fossa	15-11
Intertubercular Sulcus	19-106
Parieto-Occipital Sulcus	27-D3
Sylvian Fissure	26-49
Ventral Median Fissure	27-C1
Suprarenal Glands	10-D3,D24;21-105;
Superior Colliculi	15-16
SUTURE	
Lambdoidal	21-11
Sagittal	21-10
Squamosal	21-12
Swallowing, Position of	
Larynx and Pharynx in	20-IIA
Sylvian Fissure	26-49
T	
Tactile Body	3-4
TACTILE RESPONSES	
Tactile Responses	3-V,VI
Cold	3-D
Heat	3-F
Pain	3-A
Tickling	3-E
Touch	3-B
Traction	3-G
Two-Point Touch Discrimination	3-C
Tarsals	1-43
Tarsal Glands	2-23,29;14-12
Taste, Functional Area of Brain	26-46
TEMPORAL BONE	1-4;9-A32;19-2;21-4
Mastoid Process of	9-A7;21-5

Anatomical Feature	Chart number, bold Feature number, light
TEMPORAL BONE (Continued)	
Petrous Part of	9-A25
Styloid Process of	9-A8
Temporal Line	
Inferior	19-1
Superior	19-127
Testis	13-A17,B12;23-7a
Thalamus	15-18;27-D21
Lateral Geniculate Body of	15-8
Thoracic Nerves	21-84
Thoracic Vertebrae	1-19;21-16
Throat (Larynx with Pharynx)	20
Thrombocyte: See Platelet	
Thrush (Canadida Albicans)	20-IVB
Thymus	22-4;23-6;26-31
Thyroid	20-IIB14,III10;22-3;23-3;26-36
Tibia	1-41;19-81;21-45
TISSUE	28;29
Connective	6-D5;29
Adipose	29-5
Subcutaneous	3-IV
Areolar	29-4
Cancellous, Bone	29-11
Cartilage	
Elastic	29-9
Fibrocartilage	29-10
Hyaline	29-8
Compact Bone	29-12
Elastic	29-6
Fat	4-B10,D9
Fibrous (Dense)	29-7
Liquid, Blood	29-2
Mesenchymal	29-1
Reticular	29-3
Epithelial	28-A
Columnar	6-C8
Pseudo-Stratified (Ciliated)	28-A5
Simple	28-A4
Cuboidal	28-A3
Squamous, Simple	28-A1
Stratified	28-A2
Muscular	28-B
Cardiac	28-B5
Skeletal-Bundles	28-B2
Skeletal Cells	28-B1
Smooth Bundles of	28-B4
Smooth Cells	28-B3
Nervous	28-C
Autonomic Ganglion Cell	28-C6
Bipolar	28-C2
Multipolar	28-C3
Purkinje Cell	28-C5
Pyramidal Cell	28-C4
Pseudounipolar	28-C1
With Various Types of Neurons	28-C
Tongue	5-5; 7-29;8-B8;20-IIB5,IIB21; 26-51
Root of	20IA1,IB1
TONSIL	7-30;20-III15
Lingual	20-IA3,IB3;25-H4
Palatine	25-H3
Pharyngeal	20-IIB1;25-H2
Swollen	8-D4
Tonsilitis	20-IVA
TRACHEA	
Trachea (Windpipe)	5-12;7-25;8-A7;19-19;20-IB9,IIB13,III9; 30-E6
Bifurcation	7-13;8-E2
Cross Section of, Inflamed	8-E
Triceps	21-56
TROCHANTER	
Greater	19-59;21-43
Lesser	19-60;21-44
Trochlea	14-32
Tuber Cinereum	27-A9
TUBERCLE	
Corniculate	20-IA8,IB8
Cuneiform	20-IA7,IB7
of Epiglottis	20-IA4,IB4
TUBULES	
Collecting	10-C12
Renal	10-C5
Seminiferous	13-B11

Anatomical Feature	Chart number, bold Feature number, light
U	
ULCER	
Duodenal	**6**-A6
Peptic	**6**-D2
Ulna	**1**-26;**19**-96
Umbilical Cord	**11**-H7,K5;**12**-C6
Ureters	**10**-A10.D18;**12**-A1;**13**-A3,B1
	19-98;**21**-109
URETHRA	
External Meatus	**13**-A15;
Membranous	**13**-A10,B8
Penile	**13**-A13
Prostatic	**13**-A8
Vaginal	**12**-A10
URINARY BLADDER	
Urinary Bladder	**10**-D13;**12**-A8;**13**-A4;**19**-86;**21**-103;**31**-E12
Apex	**13**-A6c
Body	**13**-A6a
Neck	**13** A6b
UTERUS	
Uterus	**11**-J1
Corpus	**12**-A21
Endometrium	**11**-J16
Orifice of	**12**-A18
Os of, External	**11**-J12;**12**-C3
Inner	**12**-C2
Outer	**11**-J10;**12**-C3;**11**-J12
Rectouterine Pouch (of Douglas)	**12**-A20
Section, after Delivery	**12**-C
Uterus, Fallopian Tubes, and Ovaries	**11**-J
Uvula	**20**-III2
V	
Vagina	**11**-J13;**12**-C4,A11,A12
Vagus Nerve	**8**-A1,D5;**26**-21,26;**27**-A13,
	30-C1
VALVES OF THE HEART	
Aortic	**4**-A14,C1
Posterior Cusp	**4**-C7a
Right Cusp	**4**-C7b
Left Cusp	**4**-C7c
Mitral	**4**-A16,C3
Posterior	**4**-C3a
Anterior	**4**-C3b
Pulmonary	**4**-A13,C5
Anterior Cusp	**4**-C5a
Left Cusp	**4**-C5c
Right Cusp	**4**-C5b
Semilunar Cusps	
Closed	**4**-C1
Open	**4**-C2
Tricuspid (Atrio-Ventricular)	**4**-A13,A14,A27
Anterior Cusp	**4**-C8a
Medial Cusp	**4**-C8b
Posterior Cusp	**4**-C8c
Trabeculae Carnae	**4**-A25
Valves of Lymph Vessels	**24**-D
VEINS	
Arcuate	**10**-C10
Axillary	**19**-26
Basilic	**19**-35
Brachiocephalic	**4**-A3
Left	**19**-21
Right	**19**-113
Cephalic	**19**-32
Accessory	**19**-38
of Eye	**2**-7
Femoral	**19**-62,65
Lateral Circumflex	**19**-64
Gonadal	**10**-D20
Hepatic	**10**-D27
Iliac	**13**-A1;**19**-91
Interlobular, of Kidney	**10**-C7
Intestinal	**6**-C7
Jugular, External	**19**-119
Internal	**19**-20
Median Antebrachial	**19**-39
Median Cubital	**19**-36
Pulmonary	**4**-B3
Left	**4**-A11
Right	**4**-A31
Renal	**10**-A12,D22

Anatomical Feature	Chart number, bold Feature number, light
VEINS (Continued)	
Ramification of	**10**-A6
Saphenous, Great	**19**,73,74
Of Skin	**3**-19,27,28
Stellate	**10**-C4
Subclavian	**19**-22
Thyroid, Inferior	**19**-116
Vena Cava	
Inferior	**4**-A24,B6;**10**-D25;**19**-102
Superior	**4**-A4,B2;**19**-111;**24**-29;**26**-35
Venule, Skin	**3**-17
Vas Deferens	**13**-A9,B16,B2,B4,B5
VENTRICLE	
Fourth (Brain)	**15**-10;**27**-D35
Lateral (Brain)	
Anterior Horn of	**27**-B2
Inferior Horn of	**27**-B19
Posterior Horn of	**27**-B15
Left (Heart)	**4**-A15,B8
Right (Heart)	**4**-A28,D8;**7**-20
Third (Brain)	**15**-17;**27**-B21,D10
Tela Choroidea of	**27**-D12
Venule	**3**-17
Vermis	**27**-B14.D38
Vertebral Column	**26**-23
VERTEBRAE	
Cervical	**1**-9;**21**-15
Lumbar	**21**-18
Fifth Lumbar	**1**-24
Thoracic	**21**-16
Twelfth Thoracic	**1**-19
VESICLE	
Vesiculouterine Pouch	**12**-A7
Germinal	**11**-G2
Seminal	**13**-A25,B6
VESSELS: See Blood, Vessels; Lymph Vessels	
Vestibule	
of Ear	**9**-B8
Fenestra of	**9**-A11
Villus (Villi) in Development of Human Embryo	**11**-F2,H3
Intestinal Villus	**6**-C;**25**-I
Artery and Vein	**25**-I2
Digestive Disorders	**6**
VISION	**2**;**26**-12
Calcarine Sulcus	**27**-D1
Functional Area of Brain	**26**-12
Hyperopia (Farsightedness)	**2**-C
With Glasses	**2**-C41
Without Glasses	**2**-C40
Line of Comparison of Differences in Focal Plane	**2**-1A-C
Myopia (Nearsightedness)	**2**-B
With Glasses	**2**-B38
Without Glasses	**2**-B37
Normal Sight	**2**-A
Protective Mechanism of the Eye	**14**
Sight as a Function of the Brain	**15**
Visual Speech Area of Brain	**26**-9
VOCAL CORD	**7**-26;**8**-A6;**20**-IA5,IB5,IIB10;**25**-H6
Vestibular Fold	**20**-IA12,IB12
Laryngeal Polyp of	**20**-IC1
Vocal Slit	**20**
Viscera	**21**-101,109
W	
WALL	
Abdominal	**10**-D8
Orbital	**2**-A3
White Matter	**27**-C7
X	
Xiphoid Process	**1**-18;**19**-103
Y	
Yolk of Human Egg	**11**-G1,H8
Z	
Zygomatic Arch	**1**-6;**14**-10;**26**-43
Zygomatic Bone	**19**-13
Zygote	**11**-A,B,C,D
Zona Pellucida	**11**-G4